THE RAINBOW DIET

A Colorful Way to Lose Weight, Nourish Your Chakras, and Optimize Your Health and Energy

By Atari Vishnu

Copyright © 2023 by Atari Vishnu

All rights reserved.

The Rainbow Diet: A Colorful Way to Weight Loss and Optimal Health

By Atari Vishnu

Table of Contents

INTRODUCTION	1
CHAPTER 1: THE MIRACLE AND MYSTERY OF LIGHT AND COLOR	7
Color and Food	8
CHAPTER 2: THE ANCIENT WISDOM OF CHAKRAS	10
The Hidden Link Between Ancient Hindu and Ancient Hebrew Philosophies	12
The Crescendo of the Rainbow Pattern Through the Week	14
CHAPTER 3: THE SACRAMENT OF FOOD	16
Food as the Embodiment of Color	17
CHAPTER 4: HOW TO LOSE WEIGHT AND OPTIMIZE YOUR HEALTH WITH THE RAINBOW DIET	19
The Power of the Weekly Cycle of Color	20
Bringing it Together: Color, Chakras and the Week	20
CHAPTER 5: RED MONDAY: SUPPORTING THE ROOT CHAKRA	23
Ideas for a Healthful and Energetic Red Breakfast	23
Energetic Red Monday Lunch Ideas	24
Ideas for Energy-packed Red Monday dinners	25
A Shopping List of Ingredients for Red Monday	25
Transform Your Ho-Hum Fare to a Surge of Red Monday Energy	26
CHAPTER 6: ORANGE TUESDAY: SUPPORTING THE SACRAL CHAKRA	28
Ideas for a Sensual and Delicious Orange Breakfast	29
Creative Orange Tuesday Lunch Ideas	30

THE RAINBOW DIET

Orange Tuesday Creative Ideas for Dinner 30
A Shopping List of Ingredients for Orange Tuesday 31
Jump-start Orange Tuesdays 32

CHAPTER 7: YELLOW WEDNESDAY: SUPPORTING YOUR SOLAR PLEXUS CHAKRA 33

Ideas for a Powerful Yellow Breakfast 34
Yellow Wednesday Power Lunch Ideas 35
Dishes for a Powerful Yellow Wednesday Dinner 36
A Shopping List of Ingredients for Yellow Wednesday 37
Tips to Launch Yellow Wednesday 37

CHAPTER 8: GREEN THURSDAY: SUPPORTING THE HEART CHAKRA 39

Ideas for a Connected and Gracious Green Breakfast 40
Lunch Ideas for a Vibrant Green Thursday 41
Heartfelt Green Thursday Dinner Ideas 41
A Shopping List of Ingredients for Green Thursday 42
Convert Your Everyday Meals Into Powerful Green Thursday Delicacies 43

CHAPTER 9: BLUE FRIDAY: SUPPORTING THE THROAT CHAKRA 45

Ideas for an Authentic and Empathetic Blue Breakfast 46
Giving Voice to Blue Friday Lunch 47
Straightforward Blue Friday Dinner Menus 47
A Shopping List of Ingredients for Blue Friday 48
A Multitude of Blueberry Ideas 49

CHAPTER 10: INDIGO SATURDAY: SUPPORTING THE THIRD EYE CHAKRA 51

Ideas for a Breakfast to Nurture Insight and Clarity on Indigo Saturday 52
Productive Indigo Saturday Lunch Ideas 53
Indigo Saturday Dinner Ideas 53
A Shopping List of Ingredients for Indigo Saturday 54
Dynamically Launch Your Indigo Saturday 54

CHAPTER 11: VIOLET SUNDAY: SUPPORTING THE CROWN CHAKRA 56

Ideas for a Transcendent Violet Breakfast... 57
Serene Violet Sunday Lunch Ideas.. 57
Spiritual Sunday Dinners in Violet.. 58
A Shopping List of Ingredients for Violet Sunday................................... 58
Spark a Transcendent Violet Sunday.. 59

CHAPTER 12: BROWN FOR BALANCE, AND WHITE FOR SERENITY: COMPLETING THE RAINBOW 61

Brown for Balance.. 61
White for Serenity—Supporting your higher chakras with white foods 64

CHAPTER 13: BEYOND THE RAINBOW: TWO SECRETS REVEALED ABOUT WHY THE RAINBOW DIET OPTIMIZES YOUR PHYSICAL, MENTAL AND SPIRITUAL HEALTH AND HELPS YOU SUCCEED WHERE OTHER DIETS FAIL 67

Secret Number One.. 68
Secret Number Two.. 69
Why the Rainbow Diet Succeeds Where Other Diets Fail 70

CHAPTER 14: HOW YOU CAN EMBRACE THE RAINBOW DIET AND CHANGE YOUR LIFE 72

How to Begin—and Succeed at—the Rainbow Diet............................. 74

ABOUT THE AUTHOR 76

Introduction

As a child, I was entranced by colors. Before the first day of school each year, I would look forward to the day when we'd buy new crayons for my new school year. I would spend hours rearranging the colors in the box, placing them in the order of the rainbow, loving the gradual shift from dark to light, blue to green to yellow. This fascination with colors and their power has stayed with me through the years and led me to explore how color plays a role in ancient wisdom and knowledge, including chakras and energy centers.

My studies of chakras and energy centers have taught me that our bodies are wired to connect our different meridians and energy centers. These centers of energy, when balanced and functioning optimally, allow us to experience good health, vitality, and well-being. When our energy centers are blocked, we can experience a range of physical and emotional issues. But chakras are not just a philosophical idea, but are part of our anatomy. Each chakra is a bundle of nerves, connected to our glands—which produce the hormones that energize us, drive us to fight or flight, stimulate arousal, or allow us to drift off to a peaceful sleep.

This is where the Rainbow Diet comes in. The Rainbow Diet is a way to enhance our health, weight loss, and well-being by adding colorful and nutritious foods to our diets to directly support our chakras, our central nervous systems, and our hormones—and through this, our metabolism, sense of wellness, and overall health. The Rainbow Diet does not require you to be a vegetarian or follow a specific dietary plan. Rather, it is a way of thinking about the foods we eat and ensuring that we are consuming a wide variety of colorful foods that provide us with the nutrients we need to thrive. The ancient Indian spiritual and physical tradition of chakras associates the seven chakras with the seven colors of the rainbow. The Old Testament gives us our seven-day week—and nurturing the seven chakras on successive days, beginning with the red, high-energy and survival-oriented root chakra on Monday, up the spectrum toward the higher chakras, culminating with the deeply spiritual violet/white crown chakra on the restorative and restful seventh day, creates a perfect roadmap for weight loss—and physical and spiritual well-being.

Color plays a crucial role in our lives, and not just aesthetically. Each color possesses unique energy and vibrational qualities that can impact our physical, emotional, and mental well-being. This ancient knowledge is something that has been passed down for centuries, and today, we can harness it in a variety of ways, but especially through the foods we eat. Food is central to life, and our food directly affects—positively or negatively—how our bodies are able to cope with stress, tackle ambitious goals, maintain a healthy metabolism, fight off disease, and experience joy, pleasure, rest and fulfillment.

In this book, I want to introduce you to the Rainbow Diet, a way of eating that is based on the power of color and nutrition. The Rainbow Diet is not a fad or a trend - it is a way of life that has been embraced by cultures around the world for centuries. It is a way to enhance your health, support your weight loss goals, and promote overall well-being by incorporating colorful, nutritious foods into your diet in a deliberate way to create a virtuous seven-day cycle of energy, vitality, reflection and rest. The chakras are situated in a column running up your core, from the base of your spine (the root chakra) to the top of your head (the crown chakra), in a progression from survival to transcendence. The root chakra, powered and infused with the color red, is about basic energy, vitality, and general health. Beginning on a supercharged Red Monday, we focus on and nourish the root chakra to begin the week with a burst of energy. Each day we move up one chakra, and one color along the prism, nurturing and energizing each chakra in turn, until we come to the sublime Violet Sunday, in which we celebrate our connection to our highest self, stimulating restfulness, tranquility, and the culmination of our week. Reaching this climax prepares us for the burst of energy to begin the next Red Monday. The entire cycle nurtures each chakra, its associated energy and hormone center, and ensures that the entire body, stage by stage, is nourished, nurtured, energized and allowed to flourish, as we move along the entire spectrum of colors throughout the week.

The Rainbow Diet

Now, you might be thinking that this sounds like a vegetarian or vegan diet - but that's not necessarily the case. While many plant-based foods are rich in color and nutrition, the Rainbow Diet is not about eliminating certain food groups or making drastic changes to your diet. Instead, it's about incorporating a wide range of colorful foods into your meals to support your body's energy centers and promote optimal health.

Before we dive into the specifics of the Rainbow Diet, allow me to explain in greater detail the concept of chakras. Chakras are energy centers within the body that govern various physical, emotional, and mental functions. There are seven main chakras that run from the base of the spine to the crown of the head, each associated with a specific color and energy frequency:

Root Chakra (Red): The root chakra is located at the base of the spine and is associated with feelings of safety, security, and grounding. For thousands of years, the root chakra has been associated with the color red, the color associated with raw energy, vitality and power. Red foods support this chakra and promote physical energy.

Sacral Chakra (Orange): The sacral chakra is located just below the navel and is associated with creativity, sensuality, and emotional balance. The sacral chakra is tied to the color orange; orange foods support this chakra and promote emotional stability, well-being, sexual energy, and a sense of security in which creativity may flourish.

Solar Plexus Chakra (Yellow): The solar plexus chakra is located in the upper abdomen and is associated with personal power, self-confidence, and digestion. The solar plexus chakra is situated directly in your solar plexus—a critical junction of interconnected nerves located at your diaphragm, which enables your very breath. Having the "wind knocked out of you" occurs when the solar plexus chakra receives a blow and is temporarily unable to provide the energy and sustenance of pure breath. Ancient wisdom associates the color yellow with the solar plexus chakra, and yellow foods directly support this chakra and promote digestive health, breathing, and a sense of calm and equilibrium.

Heart Chakra (Green): The heart chakra is located in the center of the chest—literally at your heart—and is associated with love, compassion, and emotional balance. The center of your live-giving circulatory system, the heart chakra lies at the exact center of your vitality. Ancient wisdom associates this central chakra with the color green—no surprise, since green is the color of healthy, living plants, which supply the earth with clean air and sustenance for all plants and animals. Green foods support this chakra and promote emotional and physical health.

Throat Chakra (Blue): The throat chakra is located in the center of the neck, right below the Adam's Apple, along the vital passageways where air, nourishment and the nervous system pass between the head and the body—as well as the exact location of your critical speech organs. Philosophers have long maintained the connection between the throat chakra and the color blue; blue is accordingly associated with communication, self-expression, and creativity. Blue foods nourish and support this chakra and promote clear communication, expression, and embracing your voice and the power of using your voice to accomplish your highest aspirations.

Third Eye Chakra (Indigo): The third eye chakra is located in the center of the forehead, exactly at the seat of wisdom associated with the philosophical construct of the third eye—the eye that is not deceived by illusion or earthly distractions, but directly perceives the truth of reality. The third eye is connected to the color indigo, and is associated with intuition, perception, truth and insight. Indigo foods support this chakra and promote mental clarity, seeing through deception and distraction, and achieving true understanding.

Crown Chakra (Violet): The crown chakra, our center of highest aspiration and transcendence, is located at the top of the head. Our crown chakra is the center for spiritual connection and community, and the source of our spiritual aspiration and bonding. This highest chakra embodies the color violet (and sometimes white), and is associated with spiritual connection, consciousness, and enlightenment. Violet (and white) foods support this chakra and promote spiritual growth, connection, and transcendence.

As we delve deeper into the Rainbow Diet, we will explore the seven colors of the rainbow and the foods associated with them. We will begin on Monday, the start of the week, with the color red, which is associated with the root chakra. We will discuss the many health benefits of red foods, such as beets, tomatoes, and red peppers, and how they can help us feel grounded and energized. Moving on to Tuesday, we will focus on orange foods, which are associated with the sacral chakra. We will explore the many benefits of foods such as sweet potatoes, oranges, and carrots, and how they can help us connect with our emotions and creativity.

The Rainbow Diet

Wednesday will bring us to the color yellow and the solar plexus chakra. We will discuss the importance of foods like bananas, corn, and yellow peppers in helping us feel empowered and confident. On Thursday, we will explore the color green, which is associated with the heart chakra. We will talk about the many benefits of leafy greens, broccoli, and other green vegetables, and how they can help us feel more connected and open to love.

Friday begins the transition from the most physical elements of our beings toward the higher powers of communication, insight, and spiritual fulfillment. On Fridays we will emphasize blue foods, which are associated with the throat chakra. We will discuss the many health benefits of blueberries, blue corn, and other blue foods, and how they can help us communicate more clearly and effectively. Saturday is all about indigo, which is associated with the third eye chakra. We will explore the benefits of foods like eggplant, blackberries, and purple grapes in helping us tap into our intuition and inner wisdom. Finally, we will end the week with the color violet and the crown chakra. We will discuss the many benefits of foods like cauliflower, cabbage, and purple potatoes in helping us feel connected to the divine and our higher purpose.

We will explore how the systematic progression of our support of each chakra enables us to synchronize our journey through the week in an ideal state to face the tasks and challenges in sequence. We begin each week with a burst of raw, red energy, then move on each successive day to a more refined and nuanced energy state. In this way, we create a repeating wave, or cycle, which gets our week off to a powerful start, moves us through emotional well-being, creativity, confidence, truth and clarity, and communication—then moving to the weekend to recenter on truth, spirituality and rejuvenation. This pattern aligns your metabolism with your weekly activities, which leads to increased energy, well-being, and weight loss, since it places your body, mind and spirit in harmony with the natural cycle of your life.

In addition to the seven colors of the rainbow, we will also explore the importance of brown, white, and clear foods in our diets. These foods, although not part of the traditional rainbow spectrum, are still important in promoting balance and vitality in our bodies. We will learn how to enhance the nutrition and energetic qualities of your diet to achieve optimum health, vigor, rest, awareness, and serenity.

Through the Rainbow Diet, we will learn how to incorporate a wide variety of colorful and nutritious foods into our diets, and in turn, promote energy, stamina, health, and weight loss. So join me on this journey into the power of color and discover the many benefits of the Rainbow Diet.

Chapter 1

The Miracle and Mystery of Light and Color

Let us begin our journey with a scientific explanation of light.

Light is a form of electromagnetic radiation that travels through space in the form of an amazing and mind-bending duality of particles and waves. The basic unit of light, the photon, has both wavelike and particle-like qualities. Scientists have repeatedly shown that light can be described as either a particle or a wave, depending on how the scientist decides to detect the light in question. Light transmits energy and information throughout the universe. Photons are constantly created, absorbed, and re-emitted as light interacts with material in the universe.

The color of light that we perceive is determined by its wavelength. Different wavelengths of light correspond to different colors in the visible spectrum. For example, the longest wavelengths of the visible spectrum are red, while the shortest are violet. Other colors, such as orange, yellow, green, and blue, have wavelengths that fall between these two extremes.

But wavelength is not the only critical property of light—the other is frequency, or how many waves are encountered in a given time. Wavelength and frequency vary in an inverse relationship—i.e., the longer the wavelength, the lower the frequency, and the shorter the wavelength, the higher the frequency. Mathematically, this relationship is expressed by this equation:

$$c = \lambda \nu$$

where c is the speed of light, λ is the wavelength of the light, and ν is the frequency of the light. This equation, known as the speed of light equation, shows that the speed of light is equal to the product of the wavelength and frequency of the light.

In simpler terms, shorter wavelengths have higher frequencies, and longer wavelengths have lower frequencies. This means that blue light, which has a shorter wavelength than red light, has a higher frequency than red light.

The relationship between wavelength and frequency is important because it determines the properties of light and how it interacts with matter. The frequency of light determines the energy of the light. This means that red light has the lowest energy of light on in the visible spectrum—with orange, yellow, green, blue, indigo and violet increasing in energy. "Infrared" light means light of an even lower frequency ("infra" means "below") than red, while "ultraviolet" means light of an even higher frequency ("ultra" means "beyond") than violet. Beyond the visible spectrum, high frequency light, such as gamma rays and X-rays, have higher energies than lower frequency light, such as radio waves and microwaves.

Additionally, the wavelength of light determines how the light interacts with different materials. Some materials absorb certain wavelengths of light while reflecting others, which is why different objects have different colors. This phenomenon is the basis color and is an important aspect of many areas of science, including optics and astronomy.

When light strikes an object, the object can absorb some or all of the light's energy. This absorption causes the atoms and molecules in the object to vibrate, which in turn may cause the energy to be converted into heat, or re-emitted as light, possibly of a different wavelength/frequency. However, not all wavelengths of light are absorbed equally by all objects. Instead, different objects absorb different wavelengths of light, depending on their chemical composition and physical properties.

Color and Food

Objects, including food, modify light to take on particular properties such as color through a process known as absorption and reflection. The color of an object is determined by the wavelengths of light that are absorbed and the wavelengths that are reflected or transmitted. Red foods, or anything we see that appears red, is perceived as "red" because these objects embody and transmit the energy of the red part of the spectrum; and so on for foods or objects that we perceive as orange, yellow, green, blue, indigo or violet.

The Rainbow Diet

In the case of food, the different colors that we see are a result of the different pigments that are present in the food. For example, the red color in tomatoes comes from a pigment called lycopene, while the orange color in carrots comes from a pigment called beta-carotene. These components of food, which determine our perception of the food's color, embody the energy of the wavelength of the color we perceive. In other words, the nutritional and energetic content of food is literally described by, and embodied in, the color of the food.

This is the most basic insight of the Rainbow Diet—the energy of our food is embodied by the food's color, and by eating foods of a certain color we can ingest the energy of that color in support of the related energy centers of our bodies. A red tomato literally contains the red energy that nourishes, supports and activates our root chakra, just as purple cauliflower, with its shades of violet and white, literally contains and transmits the violet and white energy that activates our crown chakra.

While many people enjoy foods of different colors in their diets, the Rainbow Diet is transformative because it *deliberately* nourishes and energizes the energy centers of the body in a particular, systematic virtuous cycle that inevitably leads to increased health and well-being of the entire body, while leading to weight-loss, increased physical and sexual energy, creativity, vitality, communication and enlightenment. The Rainbow Diet is backed by the science of light and the ancient wisdom of the chakras in the body and the ancient wisdom of the cycle of our week—which forms the cycles of our lives.

Let us now dive deeper into the understanding of chakras passed down to us for thousands of years.

CHAPTER 2

The Ancient Wisdom of Chakras

The concept of chakras is an ancient philosophy that originated in India and has been part of the Hindu, Buddhist, and Jain spiritual traditions for thousands of years. In these ancient traditions, chakras are centers of energy that are located in different parts of the body. There are seven major chakras in the body, and each one is associated with a different color, a specific location, and a unique quality.

The seven chakras are:

Root Chakra: Located at the base of the spine, the root chakra represents our foundation and connection to the earth. It is associated with the adrenal glands, and controls the functions of elimination and survival. A balanced root chakra promotes a sense of grounding, stability, and security. Resonates with the color red.

Sacral Chakra: Located in the lower abdomen, the sacral chakra represents our creativity and sexuality. It is associated with the reproductive glands and controls sexual function and pleasure. A balanced sacral chakra promotes creativity, passion, and emotional stability. Resonates with the color orange.

Solar Plexus Chakra: Located in the upper abdomen, the solar plexus chakra represents our willpower and personal power. It is associated with the pancreas and digestive system, and controls metabolism and energy levels. A balanced solar plexus chakra promotes confidence, self-esteem, and motivation. Resonates with the color yellow.

The Rainbow Diet

Heart Chakra: Located in the center of the chest, the heart chakra represents our ability to love and connect with others. It is associated with the thymus gland and controls the immune system and circulation. A balanced heart chakra promotes compassion, forgiveness, and emotional balance. Resonates with the color green.

Throat Chakra: Located in the throat, the throat chakra represents our ability to communicate and express ourselves. It is associated with the thyroid gland and controls metabolism and communication. A balanced throat chakra promotes clear communication, self-expression, and creativity. Resonates with the color blue.

Third Eye Chakra: Located in the center of the forehead, the third eye chakra represents our intuition and spiritual insight. It is associated with the pituitary gland and controls the endocrine system and nervous system. A balanced third eye chakra promotes mental clarity, intuition, and spiritual awareness. Resonates with the color indigo.

Crown Chakra: Located at the top of the head, the crown chakra represents our connection to the divine and universal consciousness. It is associated with the pineal gland and controls the circadian rhythms and sleep patterns. A balanced crown chakra promotes spiritual awakening, enlightenment, and transcendence. Resonates with the color violet.

The health of each chakra is vital to the overall health of the body, mind, and spirit. When a chakra is blocked or imbalanced, it can manifest as physical, emotional, or spiritual symptoms, such as pain, anxiety, or a sense of disconnection. By understanding the functions and associations of each chakra, we can work to balance and strengthen them, promoting optimal health and well-being.

The philosophy of chakras was not widely accepted by the Western world until the 20th century. However, recent scientific research has provided evidence that supports the existence of these energy centers. Studies have shown that the chakras are connected to the nervous system and the endocrine system, which suggests that they play an important role in regulating various bodily functions. Likewise, modern science confirms that the chakras' locations in the body are centered in vital intersections of our nervous system—in essence, they are the transport hubs of the energy of our bodies.

In addition, the practice of yoga, which is closely connected to the philosophy of chakras, has been found to have numerous health benefits. Yoga has been shown to reduce stress, anxiety, and depression, and improve overall physical health and wellbeing. It is believed that the practice of yoga helps to balance and align the chakras, which in turn promotes overall health and wellbeing.

But now we are ready to take the next step in optimum health: supporting the chakras through choosing the right foods at the right time for optimal health and wellbeing. Each chakra is associated with a different color, and consuming foods of that color can help to balance and nourish the corresponding chakra. For example, the root chakra is associated with the color red, and consuming red foods such as tomatoes, beets, and red peppers can help to balance and strengthen this chakra. Similarly, consuming orange foods such as oranges, carrots, and sweet potatoes can help to balance the sacral chakra, which is associated with the color orange.

The philosophy of chakras offers a holistic approach to health and wellbeing that takes into account the interconnectedness of the body, mind, and spirit. By understanding the energy centers in our body and the foods that nourish them, we can achieve optimal health and vitality.

The Hidden Link Between Ancient Hindu and Ancient Hebrew Philosophies

According to ancient Hindu philosophy, the seven chakras are energy centers in our bodies that run from the base of the spine to the crown of the head, each representing different aspects of our being. Each chakra is associated with a specific color and has its own unique properties and functions. Similarly, in Ancient Hebrew culture, each day of the week was associated with a specific aspect of creation and had its own unique energy. The Book of Genesis, which describes how an omnipotent creator fashioned the universe—light and darkness, earth, water, plants, animals and man—in six days, and then rested on the seventh, or sabbath day, forms the basis of our modern week, and shapes the rhythms of our entire lives.

By aligning the ancient wisdom of the seven chakras with the days of the week, we can reinforce the natural cycle of the week and optimize the health of our bodies, minds, and spirits. The cycle of the week, beginning with the root chakra on Monday, aligns the body through the week, leading to optimal health by embracing the natural seven-day cycles of our lives. Each day

The Rainbow Diet

corresponds to a different chakra, and this cycle encourages us to nourish and support our physical, emotional, and spiritual well-being throughout the week.

On Monday, we start with the root chakra, which is associated with the color red and located at the base of the spine. This chakra is related to our survival instincts and our connection to the earth, and is associated with the adrenal glands, legs, and feet. By focusing on the root chakra on Mondays, we ground ourselves and establish a strong foundation for the rest of the week. On Mondays, we can nourish our root chakra with red foods, such as beets, tomatoes, strawberries, and red bell peppers.

Tuesday is associated with the sacral chakra, which is related to our creativity and sexuality. This chakra is associated with the color orange and located in the lower abdomen, near the reproductive organs. The sacral chakra is associated with the gonads, kidneys, and bladder. By focusing on this chakra on Tuesdays, we enhance our creativity and sense of pleasure.

Wednesday is associated with the solar plexus chakra, which is located in the upper abdomen and associated with the color yellow. This chakra is related to our personal power and self-esteem, and is associated with the pancreas, liver, and digestive system. By focusing on the solar plexus chakra on Wednesdays, we strengthen our sense of self-worth and personal power. Wednesday can be dedicated to yellow foods, such as lemons, bananas, corn, and pineapple, to stimulate our solar plexus chakra.

Thursday is associated with the heart chakra, which is located in the center of the chest and associated with the color green. This chakra is related to our ability to love and connect with others, and is associated with the heart, lungs, and circulatory system. By focusing on the heart chakra on Thursdays, we enhance our ability to connect with others and experience love and compassion. On Thursdays, we focus on green foods, such as kale, spinach, broccoli, and green apples, to nourish our heart chakra.

Friday is associated with the throat chakra, which is located in the throat and associated with the color blue. This chakra is related to our ability to communicate and express ourselves, and is associated with the thyroid, throat, and mouth. By focusing on the throat chakra on Fridays, we enhance our ability to express ourselves and communicate effectively. Fridays feature blue foods, such as blueberries, blackberries, and blue corn, to calm and balance our throat chakra.

The Rainbow Diet

Saturday is linked to the third eye chakra, which is located in the center of the forehead and associated with the color indigo. This chakra is related to our intuition and spiritual insight, and is associated with the pituitary gland, eyes, and brain. By focusing on the third eye chakra on Saturdays, we enhance our intuition and spiritual connection. On Saturdays, we can incorporate purple foods, such as grapes, eggplant, and purple cabbage, to activate our third eye chakra.

Sunday is the day to nurture the crown chakra, which is located at the top of the head and associated with the color violet or white. This chakra is related to our connection to the divine and spiritual consciousness, and is associated with the pineal gland, brain, and nervous system. By focusing on the crown chakra on Sundays, we enhance our spiritual connection and sense of oneness with the universe. On Sundays, we can nourish our crown chakra with white and/or violet foods, such as garlic, onions, mushrooms, and cauliflower (purple or white), to promote spiritual connection and higher consciousness.

By aligning our focus with the natural cycle of the week, we can optimize our health and well-being by nurturing and supporting each chakra in turn. This practice helps us to live in harmony with the natural rhythms of our lives and promotes a sense of balance and wholeness, as well as optimizing our metabolism and weight loss. By embracing the colors and energies associated with each chakra through our food choices, we can optimize our health and well-being.

The Crescendo of the Rainbow Pattern Through the Week

The Rainbow Diet is creates a powerful wave each week, starting with a burst of energy in the root chakra to nurture your connection to the earth, basic health, and survival—and then proceeding up the column of your spine each day to successively higher chakras, to culminate with the wave's crest at the crown chakra on Sunday, highlighting your highest aspirations, spirituality and transcendence. This weekly wave aligns perfectly with the work week as well—beginning with a burst of energy on Monday, then a focus on successive aspects of your life on each successive day as you move to higher frequency energy each day.

This pattern of energy not only ensures that you nurture and nourish each chakra, but also maximizes your body's optimum and natural energy cycle—and synchronizes your body's rhythms to the rhythm of the week. The

The Rainbow Diet

relationship is obvious—Monday is the start of the work and school week, demanding a commitment to energy and vitality to get the week off to a healthy and energetic start. Tuesday puts the focus on creativity and organic sexual energy. Wednesday tunes you into maximizing your personal power, confidence, and self-worth. Thursday moves the focus up the spectrum to love, compassion and community. Friday goes to the next level to focus on expression and communication. Saturday opens your third eye to intuition and guidance. And Sunday, the traditional day of rest and spirituality in the Christian tradition and in our work week, brings culminates our weekly cycle with our spiritual connection to the universe. As the ancients have passed down the millennia, this cycle attunes our bodies and spirits to the demands and goals of the week and puts us in tune with the optimum rhythm for our metabolisms and energetic cycles. This rhythmic cycle not only ensures that we attend to each chakra and facet of our beings in a profoundly harmonious pattern, but also tunes our body to optimum health, well-being, and weight loss.

Chapter 3

The Sacrament of Food

Food is literally the embodiment of its color. In addition to the energy associated with the food's color, different colored foods contain different nutrients and antioxidants that provide specific health benefits. As the most up-to-date science confirms, here are some examples of different colored foods and their nutritional benefits:

Red foods: Foods that are red in color, such as tomatoes, strawberries, and watermelon, are typically high in lycopene, an antioxidant that may help lower the risk of heart disease and certain cancers. They are also rich in vitamin C which supports the immune system and promotes skin health.

Orange foods: Foods that are orange in color, such as carrots, sweet potatoes, and oranges, are high in beta-carotene, which the body converts to vitamin A. Vitamin A is essential for healthy vision, skin, and immune function.

Yellow foods: Foods that are yellow in color, such as bananas, yellow peppers, and lemons, are rich in vitamin C, potassium, and other antioxidants that can support heart health and boost the immune system.

Green foods: Foods that are green in color, such as spinach, kale, and broccoli, are high in vitamins A, C, and K, as well as folate and iron. They are also rich in antioxidants that can protect against cancer and other diseases.

Blue Foods: Examples of blue foods include blueberries, blackberries, and blue potatoes. These foods contain anthocyanins, which are antioxidants that give them their distinctive blue color. Anthocyanins have been linked to improved cognitive function and cardiovascular health.

The Rainbow Diet

Indigo foods are include blackberries, figs, and plums. These foods typically contain high levels of polyphenols, which are antioxidants that can help to prevent inflammation and support healthy aging.

Violet foods include grapes, eggplant, and purple cauliflower. These foods contain a variety of antioxidants, including resveratrol, which has been linked to improved heart health and longevity.

White foods like cauliflower, potatoes, and mushrooms are often rich in nutrients such as fiber, potassium, and vitamin C. Examples of white foods include. These foods are often high in fiber, which can help to promote digestive health and prevent constipation. They may also contain vitamin C, which can support skin health and boost the immune system.

Brown foods are associated with the earth element and are often rich in nutrients such as fiber, magnesium, and vitamin E. They may also contain antioxidants that can help to prevent cell damage and support overall health. Examples of brown foods include whole grains, nuts, and beans. These foods are often high in fiber, which can help to promote digestive health and prevent chronic disease. They may also contain magnesium, which can support healthy bones and blood sugar control, and vitamin E, which can support healthy skin and immune function.

Food as the Embodiment of Color

But does the color of the food itself affect the nutritional value of the foods we eat? Absolutely! Consider the example of Vitamin D, and essential nutrient that our bodies need for many functions, including bone health, immune system support, and overall well-being. One of the primary ways that our bodies obtain vitamin D is through exposure to sunlight. The sunlight is absorbed by our bodies, and converted into compounds used as the energy and nourishment we need for robust health.

However, not everyone can get enough vitamin D from sunlight alone. For example, people who live in northern latitudes may not get enough sun exposure during the winter months, and people who cover their skin for religious or cultural reasons may also be at risk for vitamin D deficiency. In these cases, vitamin D supplements or foods fortified with vitamin D can be a helpful way to ensure adequate intake.

Just as vitamin D—sunlight!—can be obtained through supplements or fortified foods, other nutrients and components of light can be incorporated into foods of different colors. For example, yellow and orange fruits and vegetables are rich in beta-carotene, which is a precursor to vitamin A and also acts as an antioxidant in the body. Green leafy vegetables are high in chlorophyll, which helps to cleanse and detoxify the body. Red and purple fruits and vegetables contain anthocyanins, which are powerful antioxidants that can help to reduce inflammation and protect against chronic disease.

The color of food can also indicate its energy and nutritional components. For example, brown foods like whole grains and nuts are often high in fiber, protein, and healthy fats, which can help to support weight loss and overall health. White foods like cauliflower and mushrooms contain sulfur compounds that can help to boost the immune system and fight inflammation.

In summary, just as vitamin D can be obtained through supplements or fortified foods, foods of different colors incorporate the energy of the light itself, delivering the nutrition and nourishment of the light to our bodies and spirits through food. By incorporating a variety of colorful foods into our diets, we can support our overall health and well-being and ensure that we receive all of the essential nutrients that our bodies need.

But the Rainbow Diet is not just about achieving a balanced diet: it also ensures that we nourish our bodies through the natural order of the rainbow throughout the week to create the repeating, rhythmic wave that produces maximum health, energy and weight loss. In other words, the Rainbow Diet is not about just piling a bunch of colorful foods onto a plate—it's about structuring your diet so that you deliberately and systematically nurture your body's energy centers, **in order**, to achieve the repeating crescendo of energy, metabolism, and weight loss.

Let's dig deeper to see how it works in practice.

CHAPTER 4

How to Lose Weight and Optimize Your Health With the Rainbow Diet

The seven-day cycle of the Rainbow Diet is designed to align the body, increase metabolism, and optimize health by supporting each chakra in an ascending order with foods from the related color. The first day of the cycle, Red Monday, focuses on the root chakra and emphasizes red foods, which support grounding and stability. The next day, Orange Tuesday, focuses on the sacral chakra and emphasizes orange foods, which support creativity and pleasure.

As the week progresses, each day focuses on a different chakra and color, with foods that provide the energy and nutrition that the body needs to support that chakra. The colors and associated chakras progress from red to orange, yellow, green, blue, indigo, and finally violet on Sunday, which focuses on the crown chakra and emphasizes purple foods, which support spiritual connection and enlightenment.

This cycle aligns the body with the natural rhythms of the week, supporting physical, mental, and spiritual health. By nourishing the body with the specific foods that support each chakra, the Rainbow Diet can increase metabolism and optimize health by providing the energy and nutrition that the body needs to function at its best. Additionally, the focus on whole, colorful, nutrient-dense foods can help to promote weight loss and high energy levels.

The Rainbow Diet

The Power of the Weekly Cycle of Color

Putting your body on a seven-day cyclical pattern nourishes the body, mind, and spirit, optimizes health, and facilitates weight loss by providing a structured approach to eating and lifestyle habits. Each day of the week is associated with a specific color and chakra, and consuming foods of that color can help support and balance the related chakra. This approach promotes a balanced and varied diet, which can lead to increased nutrient intake and improved digestion.

The cycle also helps to regulate the body's natural rhythms, including sleep and metabolism. By aligning with the natural cycle of the week, the body is better able to regulate its circadian rhythms, leading to better sleep and increased metabolism. This can help with weight loss and maintenance, as well as overall health.

Furthermore, each day of the week is associated with a particular focus or intention, which aligns the mind and spirit with the physical body. For example, Monday is associated with the root chakra and the intention of grounding and stability, while Sunday is associated with the crown chakra and the intention of spiritual connection and intuition. By aligning with these intentions, individuals can enhance their overall sense of well-being and connection to themselves and the world around them.

Overall, the seven-day cyclical pattern of the Rainbow Diet provides a comprehensive approach to health and well-being, incorporating both physical and spiritual elements. By embracing this approach, individuals can optimize their health, increase metabolism, and facilitate weight loss while also promoting a deeper connection to themselves and the world around them.

Bringing it Together: Color, Chakras and the Week

Let's take a closer look at the relationship between the days of the week, the chakras associated with each day, and how using the Rainbow Diet can support not only weight loss and optimal health, but maximize performance throughout the week by emphasizing the focus on a progression of energy throughout the week, starting with the most physical and grounded chakra—the root chakra—and moving up from survival and physicality to higher forms of energy throughout the week. Nurturing each chakra in a series is important because it follows a natural progression from the most basic to the most complex needs.

The Rainbow Diet

At the base of the spine, the root chakra is the foundation of the chakra system, and it is associated with our most basic survival needs, such as food, shelter, and safety. When we nurture and balance the root chakra, we feel more grounded, secure, and connected to our physical body. The root chakra is attuned to the color red, and red foods stimulates and energizes the root chakra's wavelength.

Moving up the chakra system, the sacral chakra is associated with creativity and pleasure, the solar plexus chakra with personal power and confidence, the heart chakra with love and compassion, the throat chakra with communication and expression, the third eye chakra with intuition and insight, and the crown chakra with spiritual connection and enlightenment. These chakras are attuned to the colors orange, yellow, green, blue, indigo and violet, in that order, and receive energy and stimulation from eating foods of those colors.

By nurturing each chakra in series, we are able to build a strong foundation of physical and emotional health, which then supports our ability to explore and express our creativity, assert our personal power, give and receive love, communicate effectively, trust our intuition, and connect with a higher spiritual purpose.

Each chakra is also interconnected, so nurturing one chakra can have a positive impact on the others. For example, if we have a strong foundation in the root chakra, we are more likely to feel confident and empowered in the solar plexus chakra, and more able to express ourselves effectively in the throat chakra. By nurturing each chakra in a series, we create a holistic approach to health and wellness that supports our body, mind, and spirit.

Here's how the system works, on a weekly cycle, to maximize the health of your body, mind and spirit, moving up the ladder from survival to transcendence:

- Red Monday: Root Chakra - Energizes and supports our basic survival needs, grounding us for the week ahead.
- Orange Tuesday: Sacral Chakra - Stimulates creativity, sexuality and emotional balance.
- Yellow Wednesday: Solar Plexus Chakra - Boosts confidence, personal power and self-worth.
- Green Thursday: Heart Chakra - Promotes love, compassion, forgiveness and emotional balance.

The Rainbow Diet

- Blue Friday: Throat Chakra - Enhances communication, self-expression and authenticity.
- Indigo Saturday: Third Eye Chakra - Sharpens intuition, mental clarity and spiritual insight.
- Violet Sunday: Crown Chakra - Encourages spiritual connection inner peace and enlightenment.

Following this seven-day cycle, starting with the root chakra on Monday and progressing through the chakras toward the crown chakra on Sunday aligns the body with the natural rhythm of the week, and promotes optimal health, performance, and self-care.

Here are examples of people who have benefitted from the Rainbow Diet making real differences in their lives:

"I have been struggling with chronic fatigue, poor sleep and weight gain for the past few years. I tried different diets and exercise programs, but nothing seemed to work for me. That was until I discovered the Rainbow Diet. I followed the seven-day cycle based on supporting each chakra in an ascending order, with foods from the related color.

After just eight weeks, I lost six pounds, and I began to sleep better. I also noticed that I had more energy throughout the day, and I was able to get back to some of my favorite activities. The Rainbow Diet has truly transformed my life, and I highly recommend it to anyone who is struggling with their health and well-being."

   - Susan H., Cincinnati, Ohio

"I was skeptical about the Rainbow Diet because it sounded weird, but I decided to try it anyway. After following the diet for 18 months, I lost 26 pounds and I feel great. I will never go back to my old, unhealthy way of eating whatever random food comes in front of me. My old way of eating left me too tired to do the things I enjoy the most, like fishing, dancing, and being involved with my church."

   - Benton B., Huntsville, AL

Now let's see how to put the Rainbow Diet into practice, so you, too, can enjoy the benefits of weight loss, increased energy, and optimizing the balance of your body, mind and spirit.

Chapter 5

Red Monday: Supporting the Root Chakra

The root chakra, also known as the first chakra or Muladhara, is located at the base of the spine and is attuned to the color red. This chakra is related to our basic survival needs, such as food, shelter, and safety. The root chakra governs the organs and glands in the lower part of the body, including the kidneys, bladder, and adrenal glands.

When the root chakra is balanced, one feels grounded, secure, and confident in their ability to meet their basic needs. A balanced root chakra provides a sense of stability and helps to reduce stress and anxiety. It also helps to support physical health and wellbeing by supporting the organs and glands associated with this chakra.

Beginning the week with Red Monday optimizes the natural cycle of the week by providing a burst of energy from red foods. Red is a powerful, energizing color that is associated with the root chakra. Red foods like red peppers, strawberries, and beets, can support the root chakra and provide us with the energy we need to launch into the week with confidence, energy, and vigor. By aligning our diet and energy with the natural cycle of the week, we can optimize our health and well-being.

Ideas for a Healthful and Energetic Red Breakfast

1. Starting Red Monday with a nutritious and energy-packed breakfast is a great way to optimize the natural cycle of the week. There are many options for a healthy and delicious breakfast featuring red foods.

2. One option is a smoothie made with beets, raspberries, and Greek yogurt. Beets are rich in nitrates, which can improve blood flow and increase energy levels. Raspberries are high in fiber and antioxidants, which can help improve digestion and support overall health. Greek yogurt is an excellent source of protein and calcium, which can help build muscle and support bone health.
3. Try a red-based fruit salad packed with watermelon, apples, red grapes, red pairs and plums.
4. Another option for a Red Monday breakfast is a bowl of oatmeal topped with strawberries and almonds. Oatmeal is high in fiber and can help regulate blood sugar levels, which can keep energy levels stable throughout the day. Strawberries are packed with vitamin C, which can boost immunity and support skin health. Almonds are a great source of healthy fats, protein, and fiber, which can help you feel full and satisfied.
5. Finally, a delicious and simple Red Monday breakfast option is avocado toast topped with sliced tomatoes and a sprinkle of sea salt. Tomatoes are rich in antioxidants and vitamin C, which can boost immunity and support overall health.

Energetic Red Monday Lunch Ideas

Here are some ideas for a healthy Red Monday lunch:
1. Red lentil soup: Lentils are a great source of protein and fiber, and they're easy to cook. Simmer red lentils with onion, garlic, and a diced carrot or two until they're tender, then puree with an immersion blender until smooth. Add salt and pepper to taste, and a squeeze of lemon juice to brighten the flavor.
2. Red pepper hummus with red veggies: Make or buy a batch of hummus garnished with energetic red paprika, and serve with red pepper strips and cherry tomatoes for dipping. The veggies provide crunch and nutrition, while the hummus provides protein and healthy fats.
3. Quinoa salad with beets and feta: Cook quinoa according to package directions, then let cool. Roast diced beets until tender, then toss with the quinoa along with crumbled feta cheese and a simple vinaigrette made from olive oil and lemon juice. The beets provide a sweet earthy flavor, packed with dense energy.

The Rainbow Diet

Ideas for Energy-packed Red Monday dinners

Here are several ideas for an energy-packed Red Monday dinner:
1. Spicy beef stir-fry: Slice beef into thin strips and stir-fry with garlic, ginger, red bell pepper, red chard, onion, and spicy red sriracha hot sauce.
2. Roasted beet and red potato salad: Roast beets and red potatoes until tender, then toss with arugula, feta cheese, and a balsamic vinaigrette.
3. Tomato and red pepper soup: Sauté onions and garlic in a pot, then add canned tomatoes, roasted red peppers, vegetable broth, and spices. Blend until smooth and serve with a side salad.
4. Grilled salmon with roasted cherry tomatoes: Brush salmon fillets with olive oil and season with salt, pepper, and fresh thyme. Grill until cooked through and serve with roasted cherry tomatoes and steamed red chard.
5. Lentil and beet salad: Cook lentils according to package instructions, then toss with roasted beets, feta cheese, and a lemon vinaigrette.
6. Red lentil curry: Sauté onions and garlic in a pot, then add red lentils, red spinach, coconut milk, vegetable broth, and curry powder. Simmer until lentils are tender and serve with brown rice.

Remember to include plenty of red fruits and vegetables throughout the day to support your root chakra and optimize your health.

A Shopping List of Ingredients for Red Monday

Here are 25 red foods that can be used as ingredients for meals on Red Monday, which will support the root chakra, the lower glands, and nourish the physical body and its survival mechanisms:
1. Tomatoes
2. Red peppers
3. Beets
4. Radishes
5. Red onions
6. Pomegranates
7. Red grapefruit
8. Red cabbage
9. Strawberries
10. Raspberries
11. Cherries

12. Cranberries
13. Watermelon
14. Red apples
15. Red pears
16. Red grapes
17. Red plums
18. Red potatoes
19. Red lentils
20. Red kidney beans
21. Red quinoa
22. Red rice
23. Swiss chard
24. Red wine
25. Red spinach

To be clear, the Rainbow Diet does not require you to give up your existing diet, or make any radical changes to the way you eat. Rather, simply focus on substituting or adding the foods of the right color on the proper day—which supports your body, mind and spirit by supplying the energetic wavelength of that color directly to the target chakra through your food.

Transform Your Ho-Hum Fare to a Surge of Red Monday Energy

Here are some suggestions for how to convert your ho-hum Monday fare into a dynamic Red Monday:

1. Start your day with a nutritious smoothie that includes red fruits such as strawberries, raspberries, or cherries.
2. Use red vegetables such as red bell peppers, tomatoes, or beets in your salads and sandwiches.
3. Add some heat to your meals with red spices like paprika, cayenne pepper, or chili powder.
4. Incorporate red beans such as kidney beans or adzuki beans into your meals for a protein boost.
5. Snack on red foods like red apples, pomegranate seeds, or watermelon to satisfy your sweet tooth and boost your energy levels.
6. Enjoy a hearty Italian-style dinner featuring pasta with red sauce and a glass of red wine.

7. During your day, focus your attention on the color red as it appears around you. You can literally absorb the red-spectrum light into your body by shifting your focus to that color when it is present, which directs that energy to the corresponding root chakra, enhancing your energy and vitality in the core of the most physical aspect of your body.

Chapter 6

Orange Tuesday: Supporting the Sacral Chakra

The sacral chakra, also known as the second chakra or Swadhisthana, is located just below the navel in the lower abdomen. It is associated with the water element, the color orange, and is responsible for regulating our emotional and sexual energy.

The sacral chakra is the center of creativity, sensuality, and pleasure, and is closely tied to our emotions and relationships. It governs the reproductive system, kidneys, bladder, and lower intestines, and is responsible for the healthy flow of fluids in the body. When the sacral chakra is balanced, we are able to experience pleasure and joy in life, and have healthy emotional and sexual connections with others. We are creative, confident, and have a strong sense of self-worth. On the other hand, if the sacral chakra is blocked or imbalanced, we may experience feelings of guilt, shame, and self-doubt. We may struggle with intimacy, creativity, and pleasure in our lives. Physical symptoms of an imbalanced sacral chakra can include urinary problems, sexual dysfunction, and lower back pain.

Nurturing the sacral chakra involves engaging in activities that support emotional expression, creativity, and healthy sexuality. The sacral chakra is attuned to the color orange. Eating orange foods, such as sweet potatoes, carrots, oranges, and mangoes, can help balance the sacral chakra. Other ways to balance the sacral chakra include engaging in activities such as dancing, swimming, and practicing yoga poses that focus on the hips and pelvis. Mindfulness practices such as meditation and journaling can also be helpful in identifying and releasing emotional blocks that may be affecting the sacral chakra.

Moving from Red Monday to Orange Tuesday emphasizes a shift from the brute force of the root chakra to the more sensual and creative energy of the sacral chakra. This sequence naturally enhances productivity by subtly shifting the focus of work as one makes their way through the week. By emphasizing the sensual and creative energy of the sacral chakra on Orange Tuesday, one can unlock their creative potential and approach tasks with a fresh perspective—moving from high-energy survival-oriented Red Monday to a more refined and nuanced Orange Tuesday. This shift in energy helps individuals tap into their intuition and make decisions based on their emotional intelligence rather than pure logic. In this way, the transition from Red Monday to Orange Tuesday optimizes the natural cycle of the week by building on the foundational energy of the root chakra and gradually moving towards more refined energy associated with creativity and sensuality.

Ideas for a Sensual and Delicious Orange Breakfast

Starting Orange Tuesday with a breakfast featuring nutritious and sensual orange foods can help nurture the sacral chakra and support creativity and sensuality. Here are a few examples of healthy and energy-inducing orange breakfast options:

1. Orange and Mango Smoothie: Blend together frozen mango chunks, freshly squeezed orange juice, vanilla Greek yogurt, and a splash of almond milk for a refreshing and energizing smoothie.
2. Sweet Potato Hash: Dice sweet potatoes and cook them in a skillet with olive oil, diced onion, and bell peppers. Top with an egg or tofu scramble for a filling and nutritious breakfast. Egg yolks are full of orange energy that nurtures the sacral chakra all day.
3. Orange and Ginger Chia Pudding: Mix together chia seeds, freshly squeezed orange juice, grated ginger, and a splash of coconut milk. Let sit overnight in the fridge and top with fresh fruit in the morning for a delicious and healthy breakfast.
4. Orange and Carrot Juice: Use a juicer to make fresh orange and carrot juice for a refreshing and nutrient-packed breakfast drink.
5. Orange and Yogurt Parfait: Layer Greek yogurt, fresh orange slices, granola, and honey in a jar for a satisfying and colorful orange-based breakfast.

6. Incorporating these orange foods into your breakfast can help set the tone for a day focused on creativity and sensuality, while also providing your body with important nutrients and energy to start the day.

Creative Orange Tuesday Lunch Ideas

Moving on toward lunch, consider the following ideas:
1. Orange and arugula salad with grilled chicken: Combine arugula, sliced oranges, grilled chicken, and a sprinkle of feta cheese. Drizzle with a vinaigrette made with orange juice, olive oil, and Dijon mustard.
2. Carrot and ginger soup: Sauté chopped onions and garlic in a pot, add diced carrots and ginger, and cover with vegetable broth. Let it simmer until the carrots are soft, then blend until smooth.
3. Grilled salmon with orange glaze: Marinate salmon fillets in orange juice, olive oil, garlic, and honey. Grill the salmon and brush with more of the marinade as it cooks.
4. Orange and avocado toast: Mash ripe avocado on whole-grain toast and top with sliced oranges, a sprinkle of red pepper flakes, and a drizzle of honey.
5. Sweet potato and black bean bowl: Roast diced sweet potatoes with olive oil, salt, and chili powder. Serve over cooked quinoa with black beans with contrasting sliced oranges as a delicious and unexpected garnish.
6. To put together a healthy lunch with a minimum of work, try to meal prep as much as possible ahead of time. For example, roast sweet potatoes and cook quinoa over the weekend, so you can assemble the bowl quickly on Tuesday. Use pre-cut veggies and pre-cooked proteins if you need to save time.

Orange Tuesday Creative Ideas for Dinner

Here are some suggestions of how you might round out your Orange Tuesday with a nutritious and sensual dinner:
1. Shrimp stir-fry with orange sauce: Stir-fry shrimp with a mix of vegetables like orange bell peppers, carrots and onions. Toss in a sauce made from orange juice, soy sauce, and a touch of sesame oil. Serve over brown rice.
2. Spicy Orange-Ginger Tofu Stir-Fry: This stir-fry features crispy tofu, fresh veggies like orange peppers and carrots, and a tangy orange-ginger sauce with a kick of heat from chili flakes. Serve over ramen noodles with a mix of sesame and chili oils.

The Rainbow Diet

3. Orange chicken salad: Grill chicken breast and serve over a bed of mixed greens, topped with orange segments, sliced almonds, and a citrus vinaigrette.
4. Grilled Orange-Ginger Salmon: Marinate a fresh salmon fillet in a mixture of orange juice, grated ginger, soy sauce, and honey for about 30 minutes. Grill the salmon until cooked through and serve with a side of roasted sweet potatoes.
5. Butternut Squash and Carrot Soup: In a large pot, sauté chopped onions and garlic in olive oil until softened. Add in diced butternut squash and carrots, vegetable broth, and a pinch of cinnamon. Bring to a boil, then simmer until the vegetables are tender. Puree the soup until smooth and serve with a slice of crusty whole-grain bread.

A Shopping List of Ingredients for Orange Tuesday

1. Oranges
2. Carrots
3. Sweet potatoes
4. Pumpkin
5. Papaya
6. Mango
7. Apricots
8. Butternut squash
9. Persimmons
10. Cantaloupe
11. Orange bell peppers
12. Kumquats
13. Nectarines
14. Orange juice
15. Peach tea
16. Orange peel
17. Tangerines
18. Clementines
19. Blood oranges
20. Orange lentils
21. Orange honey
22. Orange jam

23. Orange marmalade
24. Orange carrots hummus
25. Orange salad dressing.

Jump-start Orange Tuesdays

Here are some suggestions for how to convert your ho-hum Tuesday fare into a dynamic Orange Tuesday:

1. Swap out your usual breakfast cereal for a bowl of sliced oranges, topped with a dollop of Greek yogurt and a drip of honey.
2. Pack a lunch that includes sliced carrots and orange peppers with hummus for dipping, and a side of fresh mandarin oranges.
3. Add some chopped sweet potatoes or butternut squash to your salad for lunch.
4. For dinner, cook up a stir-fry with orange bell peppers, carrots, and squash, served over brown rice.
5. Make a smoothie with frozen mango, banana, and a splash of orange juice for a refreshing and energizing breakfast.
6. Try roasted acorn squash with a sprinkle of cinnamon and maple syrup for a sweet and savory side dish.
7. Enjoy a bowl of pumpkin soup for lunch, garnished with a dollop of plain yogurt and a sprinkle of chili powder.
8. Grill up some orange-colored vegetables, like carrots and sweet potatoes, for a side dish with your dinner.
9. Make a quinoa salad with roasted beets, carrots, and oranges for a vibrant and flavorful lunch.
10. Snack on dried apricots or mango slices for a healthy and energizing snack throughout the day.

CHAPTER 7

Yellow Wednesday: Supporting your Solar Plexus Chakra

The solar plexus chakra, also known as the Manipura chakra, is located in the upper abdomen and is attuned to the color yellow. It is often referred to as the "power center" of the body, as it is responsible for our sense of personal power, self-confidence, and willpower. Nurturing the solar plexus chakra supports our physical health by regulating digestion and metabolism, and our emotional health by promoting self-esteem and self-worth.

When the solar plexus chakra is balanced and energized, we feel confident, self-assured, and in control of our lives. We are able to set boundaries and assert our needs, while also being respectful and empathetic to the needs of others. We have a strong sense of purpose and direction in life, and feel motivated to achieve our goals. Physically, a balanced solar plexus chakra supports healthy digestion, metabolism, and immune function.

On the other hand, when the solar plexus chakra is blocked, imbalanced or weakened, we may struggle with low self-esteem, lack of confidence, and indecisiveness. We may feel overwhelmed by life's challenges and unable to take action towards our goals. We may also experience digestive issues, such as constipation or diarrhea, and difficulty maintaining a healthy weight.

Nurturing the solar plexus chakra involves engaging in activities that promote self-confidence, self-worth, and self-care. This can include practicing self-affirmations, setting and achieving goals, engaging in physical exercise or activities that promote a sense of accomplishment, and engaging in mindful practices such as meditation or journaling.

Additionally, eating a diet rich in yellow foods balances and energizes the solar plexus chakra. Yellow foods, such as bananas, pineapples, yellow peppers, and turmeric, are rich in nutrients that support digestion and metabolism, such as fiber, vitamin C, and potassium. They can also promote a sense of energy and vitality, helping to boost self-confidence and motivation.

Moving from Orange Tuesday to Yellow Wednesday optimizes the natural cycle of the week by emphasizing the energy of the solar plexus chakra. The solar plexus chakra is associated with willpower, self-confidence, and personal power, and Yellow Wednesday is focused on supporting and balancing this chakra. Moving from the sensual and creative sacral chakra to the power center of the solar plexus chakra gives us a natural boost as we consolidate our creative energy into power and confidence, subtly shifting the focus of work as we make our way through the week.

Nurturing the solar plexus chakra supports the physical body by maintaining the health and vitality of the digestive system, liver, and pancreas. This chakra is also associated with mental clarity, decision-making, and confidence. When the solar plexus chakra is balanced, one may feel a sense of inner power, confidence, and direction in life.

Yellow Wednesday helps us step into our personal power and develop our willpower and confidence. This day is all about energy, focus, and motivation. By nourishing the solar plexus chakra with yellow foods, one can support their body and mind in maintaining balance and harmony.

Ideas for a Powerful Yellow Breakfast

Starting your Yellow Wednesday with a breakfast that includes yellow foods can help you tap into the power of the solar plexus chakra. Here are a few ideas for a healthy and energizing yellow breakfast:

1. Omelet with yellow bell peppers and turmeric: Whisk together some eggs and cook them in a pan with sliced yellow bell peppers. Sprinkle some turmeric on top for added flavor and a boost of anti-inflammatory properties.

2. Greek yogurt with sliced banana and honey: Top a serving of Greek yogurt with sliced banana and honey. This provides a balance of protein, healthy fats, and natural sugars to help you start your day off right.

The Rainbow Diet

3. Chia seed pudding with mango or banana: Soak chia seeds in almond milk overnight, and top with diced mango for a tropical twist or bananas for a burst of potassium and quick energy. This is a great source of fiber and healthy omega-3 fatty acids.

4. Smoothie with pineapple and ginger: Blend together frozen pineapple, almond milk, and fresh ginger for a refreshing and energizing breakfast smoothie. Pineapple is rich in vitamin C and digestive enzymes, while ginger is known for its anti-inflammatory and immune-boosting properties.

5. Quinoa breakfast bowl with roasted sweet potato: Cook quinoa according to package instructions, and top with roasted sweet potato cubes, chopped almonds, and a drizzle of maple syrup. This provides a balance of protein, complex carbs, and healthy fats to help you power through your morning.

All of these breakfast options feature yellow foods that can help support the solar plexus chakra and boost your energy levels for the day ahead.

Yellow Wednesday Power Lunch Ideas

Moving to lunch, here are five lunch ideas for Yellow Wednesday:

1. Quinoa and Chickpea Salad: Cook quinoa and mix it with chickpeas, chopped yellow bell peppers, diced cucumber, and a handful of fresh parsley. Dress the salad with olive oil, lemon juice, and salt to taste.

2. Yellow Vegetable Soup: Sauté diced onions, garlic, and ginger in olive oil until fragrant. Add diced sweet potatoes, carrots, and yellow squash to the pot and cook until tender. Puree the mixture until smooth and season with salt and pepper to taste.

3. Tuna Salad: Mix canned tuna with chopped hard-boiled eggs, diced celery, and diced yellow bell peppers. Dress with olive oil and lemon juice and serve on a bed of lettuce.

4. Yellow Lentil Curry: Cook yellow lentils in coconut milk with diced onions, garlic, and ginger until tender. Add diced sweet potatoes, carrots, and yellow bell peppers to the pot and cook until everything is tender. Serve over rice or quinoa.

5. Grilled Chicken and Yellow Pepper Wrap: Grill chicken breasts and slice them into thin strips. Spread hummus on a whole-grain wrap and top with sliced yellow bell peppers, chicken, and arugula. Roll the wrap and cut it into slices.

The Rainbow Diet

To put together a healthy lunch with a minimum of work, try to plan ahead and prep ingredients in advance. For example, you could cook a large batch of quinoa or lentils at the beginning of the week and use them in different dishes throughout the week. You could also chop vegetables ahead of time and store them in the fridge for easy use.

Dishes for a Powerful Yellow Wednesday Dinner

And here are some ideas for a delicious and powerful Yellow Wednesday dinner:

1. Yellow Curry: Cook some diced chicken or tofu in a yellow curry paste with coconut milk, onions, bell peppers, and carrots. Serve over jasmine rice.
2. Lemon Butter Chicken: Sear chicken breasts and then coat them in a lemon butter sauce made with garlic, lemon juice, and chicken broth. Serve with roasted yellow squash and zucchini.
3. Farro Stuffed Peppers: Cook farro according to package directions, then mix it with black beans, corn, diced tomatoes, and yellow bell peppers. Stuff the mixture into halved yellow bell peppers and bake until tender.
4. Spaghetti Squash with Yellow Tomato Sauce: Roast a spaghetti squash and use a fork to scrape out the "noodles." In a saucepan, sauté yellow cherry tomatoes with garlic and olive oil, and then mix in the spaghetti squash.
5. Honey Mustard Salmon: Combine honey, mustard, and soy sauce in a small bowl. Place salmon fillets in a baking dish and pour the sauce over the top. Bake until the salmon is cooked through, and serve with roasted sweet potatoes.
6. Yellow Lentil Soup: Sauté diced onions and carrots in olive oil, then add yellow lentils, vegetable broth, turmeric, cumin, and coriander. Simmer until the lentils are tender, then blend until smooth.
7. Yellow Squash and Corn Casserole: Layer sliced yellow squash and canned corn in a baking dish. Mix together mayonnaise, grated Parmesan cheese, and garlic powder, and spread over the top. Bake until bubbly and golden brown.
8. Yellow Pepper and Tomato Gazpacho: Blend yellow bell peppers, yellow tomatoes, cucumber, red onion, garlic, and olive oil until smooth. Season with salt and pepper, then chill in the refrigerator until ready to serve.

Enjoy your Yellow Wednesday dinner!

The Rainbow Diet

A Shopping List of Ingredients for Yellow Wednesday

A shopping list of Yellow Wednesday foods to energize your solar plexus chakra:

1. Lemons
2. Bananas
3. Pineapple
4. Corn
5. Yellow peppers
6. Yellow squash
7. Butternut squash
8. Yellow beets
9. Yellow lentils
10. Yellow curry
11. Turmeric
12. Mustard
13. Ginger
14. Yellowtail fish
15. Yellowfin tuna
16. Yellow heirloom tomatoes
17. Yellow watermelon
18. Yellow grapefruit
19. Mango
20. Papaya
21. Golden kiwi
22. Yellow apples
23. Yellow carrots
24. Yellow onions
25. Yellow potatoes

Tips to Launch Yellow Wednesday

Tired of eating the same thing over and over? Here are some suggestions for how to convert your dreary diet into a powerful Yellow Wednesday, energizing your Solar Plexus Chakra and juicing your willpower and self-confidence.

The Rainbow Diet

1. Add turmeric to your dishes: Turmeric is a bright yellow spice that is known for its anti-inflammatory properties. It can be added to rice, stir-fries, soups, and many other dishes.
2. Snack on yellow fruits: Snack on bananas, mangoes, pineapples, or any other yellow fruit throughout the day to get a quick boost of energy and nutrition, nourish your solar plexus chakra and energize your personal power.
3. Make a yellow smoothie: Blend together some frozen mango, pineapple, banana, and Greek yogurt for a refreshing and energizing yellow smoothie.
4. Incorporate yellow peppers into your meals: Add yellow peppers to your salads, stir-fries, or roasted vegetable dishes for a pop of color and flavor.
5. Use yellow lentils in your cooking: Yellow lentils, also known as toor dal, are a great source of protein and can be used in curries, soups, or stews.
6. Make a yellow vegetable soup: Use yellow squash, sweet potatoes, and carrots to make a delicious and nutritious vegetable soup.
7. Add yellow cheese to your meals: Use yellow cheese such as cheddar, gouda, or parmesan to add flavor and protein to your meals.
8. Try yellow rice: Make yellow rice by cooking rice with turmeric and other yellow spices for a flavorful and colorful side dish.

Chapter 8

Green Thursday: Supporting the Heart Chakra

The heart chakra, also known as Anahata in Sanskrit, is the fourth primary chakra in the human body. It is located at the center of the chest, near the heart, and is associated with the color green. This chakra is considered the bridge between the lower and upper chakras, connecting the physical and spiritual aspects of our beings. The heart chakra is responsible for our ability to love, connect, and empathize with others. It governs the heart, lungs, and circulatory system, as well as the thymus gland, which is essential for the immune system. When the heart chakra is balanced and healthy, we experience feelings of love, compassion, forgiveness, and empathy, for ourselves and others. When the heart chakra is blocked or imbalanced, it can manifest in physical symptoms such as heart problems, respiratory issues, and high blood pressure. Emotional symptoms can include feelings of isolation, fear of rejection, lack of empathy, and difficulty in connecting with others.

Green Thursday packs your diet with green food to heal and balance our heart chakra, leading to a more fulfilling and connected life. Moving from Yellow Wednesday to Green Thursday optimizes the natural cycle of the week by transitioning from Wednesday's inward focus on personal power and self-confidence to an outward emphasis on love, empathy, and connection. This sequence naturally enhances your productivity and subtly shifts the focus of your work as you make your way through the week: beginning with the brute force of red energy, moving to sensual and creative energy next, then to self-confidence, and next moving outward to love and connection with others. This sequence continues our crescendo from survival to transcendence, with nurturing the heart chakra in the heart of the week.

One of the best ways to start Green Thursday is with a breakfast featuring heart-healthy green foods. Examples of a healthful and energy-inducing green breakfast include a spinach and feta omelet, avocado toast with poached eggs, or a green smoothie made with spinach, kale, and fruit. For lunch, you can enjoy a hearty salad with leafy greens, vegetables, nuts, and seeds, topped with a light dressing. Other options include a green vegetable stir-fry or soup made with leafy greens and herbs. When it comes to dinner, you can create a variety of delicious and nourishing meals featuring green foods. Examples include grilled or roasted vegetables, green curry with vegetables and rice, and stuffed bell peppers with quinoa and greens. By incorporating green foods and drinks into your diet, you can further support your heart chakra. Examples of green foods and drinks that can energize your heart chakra and enhance your connection and love include leafy greens, green tea, kiwi, green apples, broccoli, and cucumbers.

To convert your usual Thursday fare into a dynamic Green Thursday, try adding more green vegetables and fruits to your meals, and be mindful of incorporating heart-opening practices into your day, such as meditation, deep breathing, and spending time in nature.

Ideas for a Connected and Gracious Green Breakfast

Starting your Green Thursday with a breakfast featuring nutritious and love-inspiring green foods can help nurture your heart chakra and promote feelings of love, empathy, and connection. Here are some examples of healthy and energy-inducing green breakfast options:

1. Green smoothie: Blend together spinach, kale, banana, apple, almond milk, and a dash of honey or maple syrup for a nutrient-packed and delicious smoothie.

2. Avocado toast: Mash avocado on whole-grain toast and top with sliced tomatoes, a sprinkle of sea salt, and a drizzle of olive oil.

3. Green omelet: Make an omelet with spinach, zucchini, bell peppers, and feta cheese for a satisfying and healthy breakfast.

4. Quinoa breakfast bowl: Cook quinoa and top with sautéed kale and avocado avocado for a nutritious and filling breakfast.

5. Green tea oatmeal: Cook oatmeal with green tea instead of water, and add chopped kiwi, matcha powder, and top with honey for a unique and delicious breakfast option.

Lunch Ideas for a Vibrant Green Thursday

Here are some ideas for a healthy Green Thursday lunch:

1. Green Salad: Start with a bed of leafy greens, such as spinach, arugula, or kale, and top with sliced cucumber, avocado, cherry tomatoes, and sliced almonds. Dress with olive oil and vinegar or your favorite dressing.
2. Broccoli and Cheddar Soup: Sauté chopped onion and garlic in a pot, then add chopped broccoli and vegetable broth. Simmer until the broccoli is tender, then blend until smooth. Stir in shredded cheddar cheese and season with salt and pepper.
3. Edamame and Farro Salad: Cook farro according to package instructions and let cool. Toss with cooked edamame, diced bell pepper, sliced green onion, and a dressing made from olive oil, lemon juice, and wasabi powder.
4. Greek Yogurt and Veggie Wrap: Spread Greek yogurt on a whole-grain wrap and top with sliced cucumbers, shredded carrots, sliced red onion, and a handful of mixed greens. Roll up and slice into pinwheels.
5. Green Smoothie Bowl: Blend spinach, frozen banana, almond milk, and a scoop of protein powder until smooth. Pour into a bowl and top with sliced kiwi, granola, and a drizzle of honey.
6. Grilled Veggie Sandwich: Grill sliced zucchini, eggplant, red pepper, and onion until tender. Layer the veggies on whole-grain bread with hummus, spinach, and a few slices of goat cheese.
7. Spinach and Feta Stuffed Sweet Potato: Microwave a sweet potato until tender, then slice open and stuff with sautéed spinach and crumbled feta cheese.
8. Pesto Deviled Eggs. Boil eggs, slice in half, mash the yolks with pesto, mayonnaise and salt and pepper to taste, and stuff the eggs with the delicious green filling.

Heartfelt Green Thursday Dinner Ideas

Here are ideas for heart-enriching Green Thursday dinners:

The Rainbow Diet

1. Green Salad with Grilled Chicken: Toss together mixed greens, cherry tomatoes, sliced cucumbers, sliced avocado, and grilled chicken for a delicious and nutritious dinner. Dress with a homemade vinaigrette made with olive oil, lemon juice, and wasabi powder.
2. Broiled Salmon with Asparagus: Broil salmon fillets with a bit of olive oil, salt, and pepper. Serve with roasted asparagus seasoned with garlic, lemon zest, and Parmesan cheese.
3. Spinach and Feta Stuffed Chicken Breast: Butterfly chicken breasts and stuff with a mixture of spinach, feta cheese, garlic, and breadcrumbs. Bake until cooked through and serve with spinach and garlic sauteed in olive oil.
4. Zucchini Noodles with Pesto: Spiralize zucchini into noodles and sauté in a bit of olive oil. Top with homemade pesto made with basil, garlic, pine nuts, Parmesan cheese, and olive oil.
5. Kale and White Bean Soup: Sauté diced onions, carrots, and celery until tender. Add kale, canned white beans, chicken or vegetable broth, and Italian seasoning. Simmer until the kale is tender and the flavors have melded together.
6. Veggie Stir Fry: Sauté sliced bell peppers, broccoli florets, sliced carrots, mushrooms, and diced onion in a bit of sesame oil. As the stir-fry expresses the liquid, add dry ramen noodles to absorb the liquid

A Shopping List of Ingredients for Green Thursday

Green Thursday is easy, because green foods abound. Here are 25 green foods and drinks that can energize your heart chakra and enhance your empathy and interconnection with others:

1. Spinach
2. Kale
3. Broccoli
4. Cucumber
5. Avocado
6. Green apples
7. Kiwi
8. Green grapes
9. Green bell peppers
10. Green beans
11. Artichokes
12. Brussels sprouts

13. Asparagus
14. Peas
15. Green lentils
16. Pistachios
17. Green tea
18. Matcha
19. Mint
20. Basil
21. Cilantro
22. Parsley
23. Arugula
24. Swiss chard
25. Bok choy

Convert Your Everyday Meals Into Powerful Green Thursday Delicacies

Here are some suggestions for converting your typical Thursday meals into a dynamic Green Thursday:

1. Add leafy greens to your salads and sandwiches: Try adding spinach, arugula, kale, or romaine lettuce to your lunch.
2. Swap out your regular grains for green grains: Instead of rice or quinoa, try cooking with farro, freekeh, or barley, which have a green hue and are high in fiber.
3. Add green veggies to your stir-fries: Broccoli, snow peas, and bok choy are all tasty green vegetables that can add a pop of color and nutrition to your stir-fry.
4. Make green smoothies: Blend together spinach, kale, banana, and pineapple for a sweet and refreshing green smoothie.
5. Try avocado toast for breakfast: Mash up an avocado and spread it on whole grain toast and top with sea salt and fresh-ground pepper for a nutritious and filling breakfast. Add miso paste for an exotic and delicious kick.
6. Swap out your white pasta for zucchini noodles: Spiralize zucchini into noodles and use as a base for pasta sauces for a low-carb, nutrient-packed alternative.
7. Add green herbs to your meals: Basil, parsley, and cilantro are all flavorful green herbs that can add a burst of freshness to your meals.

8. Roast green vegetables for a crispy texture: Roasting brussels sprouts, asparagus, broccoli, or green beans in the oven can give them a crispy texture and enhance their natural flavors.

CHAPTER 9

Blue Friday: Supporting the Throat Chakra

The throat chakra, or Vishuddha in Sanskrit, is the fifth chakra located at the base of the throat. It is attuned to the color blue and governs communication, self-expression, and the ability to speak one's truth. The throat chakra is connected to the thyroid gland, which is responsible for regulating metabolism and energy levels in the body.

When the throat chakra is balanced and healthy, a person is able to communicate effectively and authentically. Those with healthy throat chakras have clear and confident voices, and are able to listen actively and with empathy. A balanced throat chakra also supports creativity and self-expression in all forms, including writing, singing, and other artistic endeavors. On the other hand, when the throat chakra is blocked or unbalanced, a person may experience difficulty expressing themselves, feel unable to communicate their thoughts and feelings, or struggle to listen to others. They may also experience physical symptoms such as a sore throat, neck pain, thyroid issues, or losing their voice. Blue Friday nourishes and nurtures the throat chakra with blue fruits, vegetables and other foods, bringing this energy center into balance.

Moving from Green Thursday to Blue Friday optimizes the natural cycle of the week by emphasizing communication and truth-telling. While Green Thursday emphasizes connection and empathy, Blue Friday takes your personal relationships to the next level, putting a spotlight on clear communication, self-expression, and speaking one's truth. This shift from Thursday to Friday naturally enhances productivity by nurturing and building relationships on Thursday, then moving up a notch to a deeper level of communication and understanding. Ending the work week with this emphasis maximizes your personal power and accomplishment, and ensures that you finish the week you started with a burst of raw, red energy with emphasis on refinement and completion of the week on a higher level of relationship and community.

By putting an emphasis on communication and truth-telling, we can create more meaningful connections with others and express our thoughts and feelings in a clear and confident way. This can lead to more productive and fulfilling relationships, both personally and professionally.

As we make our way through the week, each day's focus builds upon the previous one, starting with the brute force of red energy, then moving to sensual and creative energy, self-confidence, community, love and connection, and finally wrapping up with an emphasis on speaking our truth. Overall, the natural cycle of the week allows us to gradually shift our focus and energy to different aspects of our lives, from the baseline energy of the root chakra higher through the body and the spectrum, helping us to achieve a sense of balance and harmony in our daily routines as we gradually shift the focus from survival to transcendence throughout the week.

Ideas for an Authentic and Empathetic Blue Breakfast

While there aren't many natural blue foods, there are some options that can add a pop of blue to your breakfast and help activate your throat chakra for clear communication and truth-telling on Blue Friday. Here are some ideas for a healthful blue breakfast:

1. Blueberry Smoothie: Blend together frozen blueberries, yogurt, and milk for a delicious and nutritious blue breakfast.

2. Blue Corn Tortilla Breakfast Tacos: Fill blue corn tortillas with scrambled eggs, black beans, avocado, and salsa for a savory and colorful breakfast.

3. Acai Bowl: Top frozen acai puree with blueberries, sliced banana, granola, and honey for a satisfying and antioxidant-rich breakfast.

4. Blue Spirulina Smoothie Bowl: Blend together frozen bananas, almond milk, and blue spirulina powder, and top with fresh fruit, granola, and coconut flakes.

5. Blueberry Oatmeal: Stir fresh or frozen blueberries into your oatmeal and top with nuts and honey for a comforting and nutritious breakfast.

Remember, it's not just about the color blue, but also about the nutrients that support your throat chakra, like antioxidants, vitamin C, and flavonoids, which can be found in blueberries and acai.

Giving Voice to Blue Friday Lunch

Here are some lunch ideas for Blue Friday:

1. Blueberry and goat cheese salad: Combine mixed greens, blueberries, goat cheese, sliced almonds, and a balsamic vinaigrette for a delicious and nutritious salad.
2. Tuna salad with blue corn chips: Mix canned tuna with a little bit of mayo and chopped celery for a quick and easy tuna salad. Serve with blue corn tortilla chips for a crunchy twist.
3. Blueberry and avocado sandwich: Mash avocado onto whole grain bread and top with fresh blueberries, a sprinkle of sea salt, and a spoon of honey.
4. Blue potato and kale soup: Sautee chopped kale, onion, and garlic in olive oil, then add diced blue potatoes and vegetable broth. Cook until potatoes are tender, then puree the soup until smooth.
5. Blue cheese and pear sandwich: Spread blue cheese onto whole grain bread and top with sliced pears, arugula, and a drizzle of honey.
6. Mediterranean blue hummus wrap: Spread blueberry hummus onto a whole wheat wrap and add chopped cucumber, cherry tomatoes, sliced olives, and feta cheese.
7. Blueberry and quinoa salad: Cook quinoa according to package directions, then mix with blueberries, chopped almonds, crumbled feta cheese, and a lemon vinaigrette.
8. Blue corn quesadillas: Fill blue corn tortillas with black beans, shredded cheese, diced tomatoes, and avocado. Cook in a pan until cheese is melted and tortillas are crispy.

Straightforward Blue Friday Dinner Menus

To wrap up your Blue Friday's emphasis on speaking your truth, try these dinner ideas:

The Rainbow Diet

1. Lemon garlic shrimp with blue potatoes: Sauté shrimp in a pan with garlic and lemon juice. Roast blue potatoes in the oven with olive oil and herbs.
2. Blue cheese and apple salad: Toss together mixed greens, sliced apples, walnuts, and crumbled blue cheese. Drizzle with balsamic vinaigrette.
3. Blue corn enchiladas: Fill blue corn tortillas with shredded chicken, black beans, and cheese. Bake in the oven and top with salsa and avocado.
4. Seared tuna with blueberry salsa: Sear tuna in a pan and serve with a fresh blueberry salsa made with diced red onion, cilantro, lime juice, and jalapeño.
5. Blueberry glazed pork chops: Season pork chops with salt and pepper and sear in a pan. Brush with a blueberry glaze made with blueberries, honey, balsamic vinegar, and thyme.
6. Blueberry quinoa salad: Cook quinoa and toss with blueberries, cucumber, red onion, and feta cheese. Dress with lemon vinaigrette.
7. Blueberry balsamic chicken: Season chicken with salt and pepper and sear in a pan. Drizzle with a blueberry balsamic sauce made with blueberries, balsamic vinegar, honey, and thyme.
8. Blueberry and goat cheese stuffed chicken breast: Stuff chicken breasts with a mixture of blueberries, goat cheese, and herbs. Bake in the oven and serve with a side salad.

A Shopping List of Ingredients for Blue Friday

Here are shopping list ideas for blue foods for Blue Friday:
1. Blueberries
2. Blue corn
3. Blue potatoes
4. Blue cheese
5. Blue grapefruit
6. Blue curaçao liqueur
7. Blue spirulina powder
8. Blue butterfly pea flower tea
9. Blue raspberry flavored candies or drinks
10. Blue algae supplements
11. Blueberry margarita cocktails.

The Rainbow Diet

A Multitude of Blueberry Ideas

Finally, it might seem that your choices for Blue Friday are limited. Not so! Here are suggestions for how to gravitate away from your routine diet to incorporate more blue foods and enhance your communication and truth-telling energy on Blue Friday by incorporating one of the most powerful blue foods—the humble blueberry:

1. Blueberry smoothie: Blend blueberries, almond milk, and a scoop of protein powder for a quick and energizing breakfast.
2. Blueberry muffins: Bake up a batch of blueberry muffins for a sweet and energizing snack.
3. Blueberry and yogurt parfait: Layer Greek yogurt, blueberries, and granola for a nutritious and tasty breakfast or snack.
4. Blueberry oatmeal: Add blueberries to your morning bowl of oatmeal for a delicious and energizing start to your day.
5. Blueberry and almond butter toast: Spread almond butter on toast and top with fresh blueberries for a quick and easy breakfast or snack.
6. Blueberry quinoa salad: Mix cooked quinoa with blueberries, chopped spinach, feta cheese, and a lemon vinaigrette dressing for a nutritious and filling lunch.
7. Blueberry and banana smoothie bowl: Blend frozen blueberries and banana with a splash of almond milk, then top with granola and more blueberries for a healthy and energizing breakfast.
8. Blueberry and goat cheese bruschetta: Top toasted bread with crumbled goat cheese and blueberries for a tasty and energizing snack.
9. Blueberry and feta cheese salad: Toss fresh spinach with blueberries, crumbled feta cheese, and a citrus dressing for a healthy and tasty lunch option.
10. Blueberry and kale smoothie: Blend kale, blueberries, almond milk, and banana for a nutritious and energizing breakfast or snack.
11. Blueberry and lemon pancakes: Mix fresh blueberries into pancake batter and add a squeeze of lemon juice for a tasty and energizing breakfast.
12. Blueberry and turkey wrap: Wrap sliced turkey, blueberries, and spinach in a whole wheat tortilla for a healthy and energizing lunch option.
13. Blueberry and almond butter energy balls: Mix almond butter, oats, and blueberries together, then roll into energy balls for a healthy and energizing snack.

14. Blueberry and yogurt smoothie: Blend plain Greek yogurt, blueberries, and almond milk for a healthy and filling breakfast or snack.

15. Blueberry and salmon salad: Top a bed of greens with grilled salmon, blueberries, and a lemon vinaigrette dressing for a healthy and energizing lunch option.

16. Blueberry and spinach salad: Toss spinach with blueberries, sliced almonds, and a balsamic vinaigrette dressing for a healthy and tasty lunch option.

17. Blueberry and cottage cheese bowl: Top cottage cheese with fresh blueberries and a sprinkle of cinnamon for a healthy and energizing breakfast or snack.

18. Blueberry and chia seed pudding: Mix chia seeds, almond milk, and blueberries together, then let sit in the fridge overnight for a healthy and energizing breakfast or snack.

19. Blueberry and beet smoothie: Blend beets, blueberries, and a splash of orange juice for a healthy and energizing breakfast or snack.

20. Blueberry and turkey burger: Mix ground turkey with blueberries and spices, then grill and top with avocado for a healthy and energizing dinner option.

21. Building on this list, here are other ideas to emphasize blue foods on Blue Friday:

22. Blue corn tacos: Swap out regular tacos for ones made with blue corn tortillas for lunch.

23. Blue cheese salad: Top a bed of greens with blue cheese, walnuts, and a balsamic vinaigrette dressing.

CHAPTER 10

Indigo Saturday: Supporting the Third Eye Chakra

The third eye chakra, also known as the Ajna chakra, is located in the center of the forehead, just above the eyebrows. It is associated with intuition, psychic ability, and spiritual insight. Nurturing your third eye chakra supports your body and health by promoting mental clarity, imagination, and creativity. When your third eye chakra is balanced and open, you are able to trust your intuition and make decisions with a clear mind. You may experience increased awareness, greater insight, and heightened intuition. This can help you navigate life with greater ease and confidence, as you are better able to recognize and pursue opportunities that align with your true path. Nurturing your third eye chakra can also benefit your physical health. The third eye chakra is connected to the pituitary gland, which is responsible for regulating hormones in the body. When the third eye chakra is balanced, it can help to regulate the body's hormones, which can support healthy growth and development, as well as overall wellbeing.

On the other hand, when the third eye chakra is blocked or imbalanced, it can have various negative effects on an individual's well-being. These negatives can include lack of clarity and vision, difficulty in making decisions and uncertainty about one's purpose or path in life; limited intuition and insight; a distorted perception of reality, leading to difficulties in understanding situations and people accurately; lack of imagination and creativity; headaches and migraines; poor sleep; and eye and vision sensitivity or problems.

Moving from Blue Friday to Indigo Saturday optimizes the natural cycle of the week by emphasizing your intuition and insight as you finish your work week and move into rest and relaxation for the weekend. After a week of hard work, it's important to take some time to consolidate your efforts from the week and gain insight, which sets the tone for restoration. Indigo Saturday is a perfect day to spend time in contemplation, meditation, and connecting with your inner wisdom. It is also a good day to reflect on your goals and plans for the future.

The Rainbow Diet sequence naturally enhances your productivity by starting with the brute force of red energy, through the week, and leading to an emphasis on our higher selves. Red energy is raw and powerful, but it can also be unrefined and uncontrolled. As the week progresses, we move into more subtle and refined energies, culminating in the higher vibrations of Indigo Saturday. By the end of the week, we have honed our physical, emotional, and mental energies, and are ready to tap into our spiritual energies. Subtly shifting the focus of our work as we make our way through the week helps to keep us motivated, engaged, and productive. It's like climbing a staircase, with each step building on the previous one, until we reach the top.

Ideas for a Breakfast to Nurture Insight and Clarity on Indigo Saturday

Here are a few examples of nutritious and insightful indigo breakfast options to nuture your third eye chakra:

1. Acai Bowl: Acai berries have a deep purple color and are packed with antioxidants and essential nutrients. Blend acai with frozen fruits, milk of your choice, and top with sliced fruits and nuts for a delicious and nourishing breakfast.

2. Purple Sweet Potato Hash: Sweet potatoes are a great source of fiber, vitamins, and minerals. Dice and sauté purple sweet potatoes with onions and your favorite veggies for a flavorful and filling breakfast hash.

3. Purple Smoothie: Blend frozen blueberries, blackberries, and raspberries with almond milk, spinach, and a scoop of protein powder for a nutrient-dense and refreshing breakfast smoothie.

THE RAINBOW DIET

Productive Indigo Saturday Lunch Ideas

Here are some ideas for a healthy and easy-to-prepare Indigo Saturday lunch:

1. Veggie wrap: Take a whole wheat wrap and fill it with a mix of chopped purple cabbage, red onion, carrots, and sprouts. Drizzle with a tahini dressing and roll it up.
2. Quinoa and beet salad: Cook some quinoa and mix it with chopped cooked beets, cucumber, and feta cheese. Toss with a simple vinaigrette made with olive oil, lemon juice, and honey.
3. Purple potato and kale soup: Sauté chopped onion and garlic in olive oil until soft. Add diced purple potatoes, chopped kale, and enough vegetable broth to cover the vegetables. Simmer until the potatoes are tender. Blend with an immersion blender until smooth.
4. Grilled eggplant sandwich: Cut eggplant into slices and grill them until they're tender. Layer them onto whole grain bread with roasted red peppers, goat cheese, and arugula.
5. Roasted beet and goat cheese sandwich: Slice roasted beets and layer them onto whole grain bread with goat cheese, arugula, and a drizzle of honey.

Indigo Saturday Dinner Ideas

Here are eight ideas for Indigo Saturday dinners:

1. Eggplant Parmesan: Slice eggplant into rounds, dip in egg and breadcrumbs, and bake until crispy. Layer in a baking dish with tomato sauce and mozzarella cheese, then bake until cheese is melted and bubbly.
2. Purple lentil soup: Sauté onions, carrots, and celery in a pot until tender. Add purple lentils, vegetable broth, canned tomatoes, and spices, and simmer until lentils are cooked through.
3. Purple cauliflower stir-fry: Stir-fry purple cauliflower with other colorful veggies like bell peppers, carrots, and snow peas. Add soy sauce and sesame oil for flavor. Serve over wild rice.
4. Baked salmon with blackberry sauce: Season salmon fillets with salt, pepper, and lemon juice, then bake in the oven. Serve with a sauce made from pureed blackberries, balsamic vinegar, and honey.
5. Purple potato salad: Boil purple potatoes until tender, then toss with a dressing made from Greek yogurt, Dijon mustard, lemon juice, and herbs.

6. Beet and goat cheese salad: Roast beets until tender, then slice and serve with crumbled goat cheese, arugula, and a balsamic vinaigrette.

A Shopping List of Ingredients for Indigo Saturday

Here is a shopping list of 25 indigo foods and drinks that can energize your third eye chakra and enhance your insight and intuition:

1. Beets
2. Blackberries
3. Plums
4. Purple grapes
5. Eggplant
6. Purple cabbage
7. Purple carrots
8. Purple sweet potatoes
9. Black currants
10. Elderberries
11. Concord grapes
12. Acai berries
13. Black mission figs
14. Prunes
15. Purple kale
16. Purple cauliflower
17. Purple asparagus
18. Purple corn
19. Purple rice
20. Wild rice
21. Purple barley
22. Purple lentils
23. Black beans
24. Hibiscus tea
25. Concord grape juice.

Dynamically Launch Your Indigo Saturday

Finally, we end with some suggestions for how to convert your standard fare into a dynamic Indigo Saturday:

The Rainbow Diet

1. Incorporate indigo fruits and vegetables such as beets, purple potatoes, blackberries, eggplant, and purple cabbage into your meals.
2. Add herbs and spices known to promote intuition and insight such as lavender, rosemary, and sage to your meals.
3. Start your day with hibiscus tea. You can also make a delicious hibiscus water by boiling hibiscus flowers, draining the liquid, adding sugar, and diluting to taste.
4. Substitute the purple version of your favorite fresh foods: purple potatoes, purple rice, purple corn, purple cauliflower, purple barley and lentils, purple asparagus and black beans are all delicious alternatives to the "standard" counterparts.

THE RAINBOW DIET

CHAPTER 11

Violet Sunday: Supporting the Crown Chakra

The crown chakra, or Sahasrara in Sanskrit, is the seventh and highest chakra in the body's energy system. It is located at the top of the head and is associated with the colors violet and white. The crown chakra is connected to our sense of connection to the divine, spiritual enlightenment, and universal consciousness.

When the crown chakra is balanced and healthy, we experience a deep sense of inner peace, connection to something greater than ourselves, and an understanding of the interconnectedness of all things. We may also feel a strong sense of purpose and direction in life, as well as heightened intuition and spiritual awareness. Releasing attachment to material possessions and worldly concerns, and focusing on cultivating a sense of inner peace and spiritual connection. Physical symptoms of an imbalanced crown chakra may include headaches, migraines, and sensitivity to light. Mental and emotional symptoms may include feelings of disconnection, depression, and confusion. Nurturing the crown chakra can support overall health and well-being by helping us to cultivate a deeper sense of purpose and meaning in life, and a greater understanding of the interconnectedness of all things. It can also support greater mental and emotional balance, as well as physical health.

Moving from Indigo Saturday to Violet Sunday completes the natural cycle of the week by emphasizing enlightenment and purpose, leading to a day of serenity and inner peace. This sequence naturally enhances restfulness and serenity, capping off a week beginning with hard-charging Red Monday with a serene and calming Violet Sunday—preparing the body, mind and spirit to begin the cycle anew the next day. A day nurturing the crown chakra supports overall health and well-being, including mental clarity, deep relaxation, and a sense of purpose.

The crown chakra is associated with the color violet or purple (and also white—as discussed in a later chapter), and eating foods that are purple or violet can help balance and energize this chakra. These foods include purple grapes, plums, berries, figs, eggplants, purple cabbage, and purple cauliflower. Drinking beverages such as grape juice, red wine, and herbal teas made with lavender or violet flowers can also help to balance the crown chakra.

Ideas for a Transcendent Violet Breakfast

Starting your Violet Sunday with a nutritious breakfast featuring violet, purple and white foods can help balance and energize your crown chakra. Here are a few examples of healthful and energy-inducing breakfast options:

1. Purple smoothie bowl: Blend together frozen berries, banana, almond milk, and your favorite protein powder.
2. Acai bowl: Blend together frozen acai, banana, and almond milk, and top with sliced fruit, nuts, and seeds.
3. Purple sweet potato toast: Slice and toast a purple sweet potato, and top with almond butter, chia seeds, and fresh berries.
4. Overnight oats with blueberries: Mix together oats, almond milk, blueberries, chia seeds, and maple syrup, and let sit overnight. In the morning, top with nuts, seeds, and fresh berries.
5. Chia seed pudding: Mix together chia seeds, almond milk, vanilla extract, and maple syrup, and let sit in the fridge overnight. In the morning, top with fresh berries and nuts.
6. Greek yogurt parfait: Layer Greek yogurt, sliced banana, blackberries, and granola in a glass, and top with honey.

Serene Violet Sunday Lunch Ideas

Here are some lunch ideas for Violet Sunday that are easy to prepare:
1. Quinoa and Chickpea and Purple Onion Salad: Cook quinoa, add in chickpeas, diced purple onion, chopped parsley, and a dressing made with olive oil, lemon juice, and garlic.

2. Purple Sweet Potato Soup: Saute diced onions and garlic in olive oil, add diced purple sweet potatoes and vegetable broth, and simmer until the sweet potatoes are tender. Puree the soup and season with salt and pepper.

3. Grilled Eggplant Sandwich: Slice eggplant, brush with olive oil, and grill until tender. Layer grilled eggplant on whole grain bread with hummus, sliced tomatoes, and fresh spinach leaves.

4. White Bean and Kale Salad: Drain and rinse a can of white beans, mix with chopped kale, sliced cherry tomatoes, diced purple onion, and a dressing made with olive oil, lemon juice, and Dijon mustard.

Spiritual Sunday Dinners in Violet

Here are here are eight ideas for Violet Sunday dinners that emphasize purple/violet foods:

1. Eggplant Parmesan: This classic Italian dish features breaded and fried eggplant slices smothered in tomato sauce and melted mozzarella cheese.

2. Beet and Feta Salad: Roasted beets and crumbled feta cheese are tossed with fresh greens and a balsamic vinaigrette for a flavorful and colorful salad.

3. Purple Sweet Potato Curry: This spicy and flavorful curry features purple sweet potatoes, coconut milk, and a variety of fragrant spices.

4. Lavender and Honey Glazed Pork Tenderloin: Pork tenderloin is coated in a sweet and savory glaze made with lavender and honey, then roasted to tender perfection.

5. Blackberry Farro Salad: Fresh blackberries, cooked farro, and tangy feta cheese are tossed with a simple vinaigrette for a refreshing and nutritious salad.

6. Purple Cauliflower Soup: Roasted purple cauliflower is blended with cream and chicken broth to create a rich and flavorful soup.

7. Blackberry and Brie Tart: This elegant tart features a buttery pastry crust filled with creamy brie cheese and topped with fresh blackberries.

8. Purple Cabbage Slaw: Shredded purple cabbage is tossed with a tangy vinaigrette and fresh herbs for a colorful and refreshing side dish.

A Shopping List of Ingredients for Violet Sunday

Here is a list of 25 violet/purple foods and drinks that can energize your crown chakra for your shopping list:

The Rainbow Diet

1. Purple grapes
2. Purple cabbage
3. Eggplant
4. Purple carrots
5. Blackberries
6. Blueberries
7. Black currants
8. Concord grapes
9. Plums
10. Prunes
11. Figs
12. Raisins
13. Acai berries
14. Elderberries
15. Purple passionfruit
16. Purple sweet potato
17. Purple yam
18. Lavender tea
19. Hibiscus tea
20. Blackcurrant tea
21. Grape juice
22. Beetroot juice
23. Purple corn
24. Purple cauliflower
25. Purple asparagus

These foods are not only beautiful, but also full of antioxidants, vitamins, and minerals that can support your overall health and wellbeing.

Spark a Transcendent Violet Sunday

Here are some suggestions for how to convert your regular meals into a dynamic and spiritual Violet Sunday:

1. Set a beautiful table: Use a tablecloth or placemats in shades of violet and white, and add some fresh flowers in the same colors as a centerpiece.
2. Create a serene atmosphere: Light some candles or incense, play some relaxing music, and dim the lights.

3. Use violet and white ingredients: Choose foods that are naturally violet or white, such as beets, purple cabbage, purple potatoes, white beans, cauliflower, onions, garlic, and mushrooms.
4. Experiment with spices: Add some violet and white spices to your dishes, such as lavender, thyme, and rosemary.
5. Make a vibrant smoothie: Blend together some blueberries, blackberries, banana, yogurt, and a splash of almond milk to make a delicious and nutritious purple smoothie.
6. Serve a colorful salad: Combine purple cabbage, sliced beets, and feta cheese on a bed of mixed greens for a colorful and flavorful salad.
7. Make a hearty soup: Use white beans, purple cauliflower, and leeks to make a creamy and satisfying soup.
8. Cook up a colorful main course: Try making a roasted vegetable medley with purple potatoes, cauliflower, and onions, or a white fish with a side of garlic sautéed mushrooms.
9. End on a sweet note: Finish your meal with a dessert featuring violet or white ingredients, such as a lavender-infused panna cotta or a coconut macaroon.

Part of nurturing your crown chakra is the enjoyment of the process of creating a special meal and to savor the flavors and colors of the food you're preparing. This is especially important on Violet Sunday, a day focused on energizing your crown chakra, the center of inner spiritual peace and long-term goals.

Chapter 12

Brown for Balance, and White for Serenity: Completing the Rainbow

The Rainbow Diet emphasizes the colorful foods that most frequently come from the fruit, roots and leaves of plants. These foods form the core of the Rainbow Diet—but the Rainbow Diet does not exclude other foods. Indeed, two other broad categories of foods, brown and white, round out the Rainbow Diet and ensure a wholesome and maximally nourishing diet.

Brown for Balance

Brown foods like grains, seeds and nuts, as well as meat and other animal products, compliment the Rainbow Diet by adding protein and energy into your daily fare. Here are some examples of brown foods and their nutritional benefits:

1. Nuts (almonds, walnuts, pecans, etc.): rich in healthy fats, protein, fiber, vitamins, and minerals, which can help improve heart health, digestion, and brain function.
2. Seeds (flaxseeds, sunflower seeds, sesame seeds, etc.): rich in healthy fats, protein, fiber, vitamins, and minerals, which can help lower inflammation, regulate blood sugar levels, and support bone health.

The Rainbow Diet

3. Whole grains (brown rice, quinoa, whole wheat, etc.): rich in complex carbohydrates, fiber, vitamins, and minerals, which can help lower the risk of chronic diseases, promote satiety, and support gut health.
4. Legumes (beans, lentils, chickpeas, etc.): rich in plant-based protein, fiber, vitamins, and minerals, which can help lower cholesterol levels, regulate blood sugar levels, and improve gut health.
5. Meat (beef, pork, chicken, etc.): rich in protein, iron, zinc, and B vitamins, which can help build and repair tissues, support immune function, and provide energy.
6. Fish (salmon, tuna, mackerel, etc.): rich in omega-3 fatty acids, protein, vitamins, and minerals, which can help lower inflammation, improve heart health, and support brain function.

Overall, incorporating a variety of brown foods into the Rainbow Diet can provide numerous health benefits, as they are often rich in essential nutrients. Whole grains, and nuts are forms of highly-nutritious brown foods, are a great addition to any balanced and healthy diet. They are high in protein, healthy fats, fiber, vitamins, and minerals, which can provide a wide range of health benefits. Fiber promotes healthy digestion, lowers cholesterol levels, and helps in maintaining a healthy weight. Protein is essential for building and repairing tissues, and healthy fats are important for brain health and reducing inflammation. Vitamins and minerals in brown foods help in maintaining healthy bones, skin, and hair. Brown foods also provide a sense of satiety and help in reducing overall calorie intake. This is because they are high in fiber and healthy fats, which take longer to digest, keeping you feeling full for longer periods.

Using brown foods in your diet can help in reducing the risk of chronic diseases such as heart disease, type 2 diabetes, and certain types of cancer. Nuts, in particular, are high in monounsaturated and polyunsaturated fats, which are heart-healthy fats that can help in reducing the risk of heart disease. Finally, incorporating brown foods into your Rainbow Diet add variety and depth to your meals, which can make it more enjoyable and sustainable in the long term.

Brown foods frequently form the base of meals in the Rainbow Diet—like oatmeal, which can be eaten with added strawberries, oranges, bananas, kiwi, blueberries, acai berries, or blackberries, to create any day's rainbow breakfast. So don't worry if the rainbow color is an accent to the meal, rather than the core of the meal. Brown foods may be used to augment or complement the day's color, and you do not need to give up on nutritious and delicious brown foods to get the most out of the Rainbow Diet.

Here are some brown foods to enhance and compliment the Rainbow Diet:

1. Almonds: Rich in vitamin E and magnesium, and a good source of healthy fats and protein.
2. Walnuts: High in omega-3 fatty acids, antioxidants, and fiber.
3. Cashews: Contain healthy fats, protein, and minerals such as copper and zinc.
4. Hazelnuts: A good source of vitamin E, magnesium, and fiber.
5. Brazil nuts: Rich in selenium, a mineral important for thyroid function and immune system health.
6. Pecans: High in antioxidants and minerals such as zinc and magnesium.
7. Macadamia nuts: Rich in healthy fats, fiber, and minerals such as iron and manganese.
8. Peanut butter: High in protein and healthy fats, and a good source of vitamin E and magnesium.
9. Pistachios: A good source of protein, fiber, and healthy fats, as well as minerals such as potassium and phosphorus.
10. Chestnuts: A low-fat nut high in vitamin C, fiber, and antioxidants.
11. Lentils: Rich in protein, fiber, and minerals such as iron and folate.
12. Farro: A highly nutritious grain that is an excellent and source of fiber, protein, and several essential minerals such as magnesium and iron. It is also rich in antioxidants and contains vitamins B and E. Due to its high fiber content, farro promotes digestive health and can help regulate blood sugar levels.
13. Quinoa: A complete protein source, high in fiber, and a good source of minerals such as magnesium and manganese.
14. Brown rice: High in fiber and minerals such as selenium and manganese.
15. Whole grain bread: A good source of fiber and essential nutrients such as iron and B vitamins.
16. Oats: High in soluble fiber, which can lower cholesterol levels, and a good source of minerals such as zinc and magnesium.
17. Chia seeds: Rich in omega-3 fatty acids, fiber, and minerals such as calcium and magnesium. Often has an indigo or violet hue, and is perfect for Indigo Saturday or Violet Sunday, but a good compliment to any day's meal.

18. Flax seeds: High in omega-3 fatty acids, fiber, and antioxidants.
19. Sesame seeds: A good source of healthy fats and minerals such as copper and magnesium.
20. Pumpkin seeds: High in protein, healthy fats, and minerals such as zinc and magnesium.
21. Beef: A good source of protein, iron, and other important nutrients.
22. Chicken: High in protein, low in fat, and a good source of vitamins and minerals.
23. Turkey: Rich in protein and a good source of vitamins and minerals such as selenium and vitamin B6.
24. Pork: High in protein, iron, and other important nutrients.
25. Salmon: A rich source of omega-3 fatty acids and protein, as well as minerals such as selenium and potassium.

White for Serenity—Supporting your higher chakras with white foods

White and clear foods, such as fruits, vegetables, and teas, are associated with the crown and upper chakras, but can also compliment and fill out any meal. These foods promote relaxation, inner peace, and spiritual growth. They are often consumed during meditation and other spiritual practices to support the higher chakras and facilitate a deeper connection with the divine. White and clear foods are also known for their cleansing properties. They are often used in detox and purification diets, as they help to eliminate toxins and support the body's natural healing processes. Many white and clear foods are high in antioxidants, which can help to reduce inflammation and support overall health

Examples of white and clear foods include these:
1. Cauliflower - Rich in fiber, vitamin C, and antioxidants.
2. Garlic - Contains compounds that have medicinal properties and can boost the immune system.
3. Coconut - Rich in medium-chain triglycerides (MCTs) that can help with weight loss and improve brain function.
4. White beans - A good source of protein, fiber, and minerals such as iron and potassium.
5. Tofu - A great source of protein, iron, and calcium.
6. White fish - Low in fat and calories, high in protein, and a good source of omega-3 fatty acids.

The Rainbow Diet

7. Greek yogurt - High in protein and calcium, and can help promote a healthy gut microbiome.
8. White mushrooms - Low in calories and high in antioxidants and B vitamins.
9. Jicama - A good source of fiber, vitamin C, and potassium.
10. Turnips - Low in calories and high in fiber, vitamin C, and potassium.
11. White asparagus - High in vitamin C and antioxidants.
12. Parsnips - High in fiber and potassium, and a good source of vitamin C and folate.
13. White onions - Rich in antioxidants and can help reduce inflammation.
14. Ginger - Can help relieve nausea, pain, and inflammation.
15. White tea - High in antioxidants and may help with weight loss and heart health.
16. Popcorn - High in fiber and antioxidants, and can be a healthy and low-calorie snack. Try seasoning with nutritional yeast instead of butter.
17. Pears - A good source of fiber, vitamin C, and antioxidants.
18. Apples - High in fiber and antioxidants, and can help reduce the risk of heart disease.
19. White potatoes - High in potassium and vitamin C, and can be a healthy addition to a balanced diet.
20. White rice - A good source of carbohydrates and can be a healthy addition to a balanced diet when consumed in moderation.
21. Coconut water - Rich in potassium and electrolytes, and can help hydrate the body.
22. Cauliflower rice - A low-carbohydrate alternative to traditional rice, high in fiber and antioxidants. Cauliflower rice is made by cutting cauliflower into rice-sized pieces—or you can buy it at the grocery store.
23. White corn - A good source of fiber and antioxidants, and can be a healthy addition to a balanced diet.
24. White nectarines - High in vitamin C and antioxidants.
25. White peaches - High in fiber and antioxidants, and can help support healthy skin.

Overall, incorporating white and clear foods into your diet can help to promote relaxation, support the higher chakras, and promote overall health and well-being. Especially on Violet Sunday, white and clear foods may be emphasized in addition to or instead of violet foods, because the crown chakra is also associated with the color white.

Here are some suggestions for breakfasts emphasizing white foods:
1. Greek yogurt with sliced bananas, walnuts, and a spoon of honey.
2. Overnight oats made with almond milk, chia seeds, vanilla extract. This nutritious and delicious breakfast can be the basis of any day of the week by adding fruit of the day's color.
3. Scrambled eggs with sautéed mushrooms and jack or white cheddar cheese.
4. Smoothie made with almond milk, frozen banana, and a scoop of vanilla protein powder. Again, smoothies may be the basis of any day's breakfast simply by adding fruit of the day's rainbow color.
5. Whole wheat bagel with cream cheese, with or without sliced smoked salmon.
6. Cottage cheese with almond slices, and a sprinkle of cinnamon.

For lunch, try these white-based dishes:
1. Chicken salad made with cooked chicken breast, diced apples, sliced almonds, and a creamy dressing made with Greek yogurt and Dijon mustard.
2. Quinoa or rice and vegetable stir-fry with tofu and a soy-ginger sauce.
3. Turkey and avocado wrap made with a whole wheat tortilla, sliced turkey breast, avocado, and hummus.
4. Vegetable soup with a side of whole grain bread or crackers and sliced cheese.
5. Chickpea and vegetable salad with a lemon vinaigrette dressing.
6. Shrimp and vegetable stir-fry with soba noodles and a spicy peanut sauce.
7. Grilled chicken and vegetable skewers with a side of couscous salad.

Try these white-food based dinner ideas:
1. Baked salmon with a side of roasted cauliflower and mashed potatoes (or sweet potatoes).
2. Grilled chicken breast with a side of roasted garlic mashed potatoes.
3. Pan-seared scallops with a side of sautéed mushrooms.
4. Grilled shrimp skewers with a side of brown rice and roasted Brussels sprouts.
5. Pork tenderloin with a side of roasted parsnips and mashed potatoes.
6. Baked tilapia with a side of quinoa and roasted carrots.

CHAPTER 13

Beyond the Rainbow: Two Secrets Revealed about Why the Rainbow Diet Optimizes your Physical, Mental and Spiritual Health and Helps You Succeed Where Other Diets Fail

The Rainbow Diet is not about eliminating other foods from your diet but rather adding more colorful and nutrient-dense foods to it. The Rainbow Diet does not require calorie-counting, eliminating foods you love, giving up alcohol or sweets, or coupling your food with a complicated exercise regimen. Rather, by focusing on the foods of the day's color, you ensure that you are getting a variety of nutrients that are essential for your body and mind to function optimally. The Rainbow Diet consistently leads to weight loss, higher energy, and optimal health by nurturing the chakras and putting your body on an optimal seven-day cycle that aligns your week with care for each chakra in turn. This cycle creates a virtual, wave-shaped pattern beginning with the forceful, blunt red energy to nurture your root chakra on Monday, then progressing one by one to higher vibrations, refinement, and transcendence as the week progresses.

But *why* does emphasis on foods of particular colors on successive days produce such a profound change in the well-being of those who practice it? Now it is time to reveal two "secrets" that explain the Rainbow Diet's consistent success.

Secret Number One

The Rainbow Diet will naturally, and painlessly, replace a significant portion of an unhealthy diet with nutritious, fresh, vitamin-packed foods, while putting your body into alignment with the world you live in.

As mentioned earlier, colorful foods almost always come from the fruit, roots and leaves of plants. Plants receive their energy directly from sunlight, and transform that pure, full-spectrum energy directly into the rainbow-hued foods that nurture your chakras, your body, and your spirit.

When you embark on the Rainbow Diet, even if you start with just adding a touch of color to your existing fare, you will automatically, and without any pain or extra work, *displace* at least a portion of your meals with the most healthful, vibrant, and nourishing food available. As you embrace the Rainbow Diet and incorporate it more and more into your life, the quantity of high-value, nutritious and delicious rainbow-colored food will become a larger and larger part of your diet—leading to enormous benefits to your energy, health and well-being.

While it is true that a less systematic diet—replacing a fried side dish with a fresh green salad every day, for example—also replaces less nutritious foods with more nutrition, the Rainbow Diet also directly supports your chakras and your energy in a way that has been studied and practiced for thousands of years. The cyclic focus on one chakra per day, beginning with the root chakra and moving up one per day to reach the crown chakra on Sunday, ensures that your body and your energy is supported systematically, holistically, and completely. Since colored food literally transmits the energy of the color of the food directly into your body, you can ensure that your body's energy centers and organs are *all* nourished, and that your body does not fall out of balance by emphasizing certain elements while neglecting others.

Finally, the deliberate alignment of your week with your body's needs ensures that you will receive the nourishment and care you need *when you need*

The Rainbow Diet

it. Many people complain of a lack of energy on Monday, and have trouble getting their week off to a productive start. The Rainbow Diet directly addresses and remedies this common shortcoming, by rushing the most energetic, bright red foods directly to the body to give the burst of energy needed to get the week off to a good start. Following the Rainbow Diet through the spectrum and up the chakras follows and amplifies the body's natural biorhythms to emphasize creativity and sensuality, self-confidence and willpower, community and bonding, truth-telling, intuition, and finally our highest aspirations, we move naturally from survival to transcendence, neglecting nothing and nurturing all aspects of our lives. This is all made possible simply by adding the energy of our food to our body's natural intelligence and direction. The virtuous cycle of energizing our body's basic nature inevitably leads to greater health.

Secret Number Two

Practicing the Rainbow Diet not only provides health benefits from the foods you eat *but also through the awareness it brings to your entire being*. By focusing on the chakras and the energy centers in the body, the Rainbow Diet encourages mindfulness and self-care. The chakras are not only affected by the food you eat, but also by your thoughts, emotions, and environment. By practicing the Rainbow Diet, you become more aware of the connection between your body, mind, and spirit, and can take steps to bring these aspects into balance.

The Rainbow Diet also emphasizes the natural cycle of the week, starting with the energetic and grounding red foods of Monday and progressing through the colors to the serene and spiritual violet, white and clear foods of Sunday. This progression supports a balanced and holistic approach to nutrition and self-care, and ensures that you are mindful of each element of your being, in its proper sequence in your body and in your life.

Exercise and other practices that support the chakras and holistic health can also be incorporated into a healthy lifestyle. Yoga and meditation are excellent practices that can help balance and open the chakras, reduce stress, and improve overall health. Other practices like acupuncture, massage, and aromatherapy can also be beneficial for holistic health. But like the Rainbow Diet, the benefit of yoga, for example, goes far beyond the flexibility and strength you build up by practicing the different poses. Instead, the *practice* of yoga leads to greater awareness and self-care, and mindfulness of how care for your body produces benefits for the body, mind and spirit.

The same is true for the Rainbow Diet—with the exception that food is *elemental* to our daily lives. Whether or not you make the time to visit the yoga studio or carve out 30 minutes for meditation, we all eat, several times, every day. By incorporating mindfulness of our chakras, the cycle of our lives throughout the week, and by nurturing our chakras and our spirits consistently and repeatedly, every day of the week, we achieve a whole far greater than simply the sum of the food we consume.

Why the Rainbow Diet Succeeds Where Other Diets Fail

Many diets emphasize the need for practices outside the diet itself. Many diet recommendations emphasize that to succeed you must focus on external factors like these:

1. Set realistic goals: Start by setting small, achievable goals for your diet and exercise routines. Gradually increase your goals as you build your strength and endurance.

2. Listen to your body: Pay attention to your body's signals, and adjust your diet and exercise routine accordingly. If you're feeling fatigued, take a rest day or modify your workout. If certain foods don't agree with you, find alternatives that work better for your body.

3. Incorporate mindfulness practices: Practices such as meditation, yoga, and deep breathing can help you manage stress and maintain a positive outlook.

4. Stay hydrated: Drinking enough water is crucial for overall health, including maintaining healthy skin, aiding digestion, and regulating body temperature.

5. Get enough sleep: Quality sleep is essential for physical and mental health. Aim for at least 7-8 hours of sleep each night.

6. Connect with others: Building and maintaining meaningful relationships can provide social support, which is important for emotional well-being.

With the Rainbow Diet, these external practices are incorporated directly into the Rainbow Diet itself. It is impossible to prepare rainbow-colored foods on a particular day to nourish a particular chakra without simultaneously—and without any extra effort—obtaining the benefits of these external practices that are encouraged by other regimens. Deliberately and mindfully eating nourishing and energetic foods naturally sets goals, encourages mindfulness of your body, acts as its own mindfulness practice, encourages hydration and sleep, and focuses your awareness on your connection to your community and loved ones—especially on Green Thursday, when every one of your meals directly supports your connection and empathy with others at the heart of the week.

These secrets make the Rainbow Diet the most powerful and deliberate way to nourish your body, mind and spirit in an easy, intuitive, and foolproof way. The Rainbow Diet explains why so many people over the millennia have embraced and thrived on the Rainbow Diet. So please enjoy the energy, connection and serenity that is yours by simply eating foods that align your body with the spectrum of colors that surrounds and permeates us—and the cycles of the week handed down to us through spiritual leaders for millennia.

CHAPTER 14

How You Can Embrace the Rainbow Diet and Change Your Life

" Nine months after embracing the Rainbow Diet, I have experienced a true change in my life. Before adopting this holistic approach to nutrition, I was constantly battling low energy, mood swings, and a lack of focus. I came across the Rainbow Diet. Even though I had never heard of chakras, I decided I had nothing to lose by giving it a try.

From the moment I started nourishing my chakras each day with the right color of healthy foods, I noticed a remarkable difference. My energy levels soared, and my mind became clearer than ever before. And I immediately loved the delicious and fun flavors I based my food around. Not only did my meals become visually appealing and delicious, but I found myself feeling more satisfied and content after each one. The Rainbow Diet opened up a world of flavors and textures that I had never explored before, making each day a delightful culinary adventure—and it pushed me to become more creative and attuned to my food.

As the months went by, the positive changes became even more apparent. I reached a healthy and stable weight effortlessly, and my body, self-image, and confidence improved. The Rainbow Diet didn't just enhance my physical health; it also had a profound impact on my mental and emotional well-being. I felt a renewed sense of balance, joy, and connection with my body and the world around me. The journey I've embarked on with the Rainbow Diet has been so transformative that I can't help but share my experience with others, inspiring them to embark on their own path towards vibrant and holistic health.

In just nine months, the Rainbow Diet has empowered me to live a truly colorful and fulfilling life. It has been a journey of self-discovery, self-care, and self-love. I am grateful for the positive changes it has brought into my life, and I look forward to continuing this vibrant and nourishing lifestyle for years to come."

—Carol M., Boston, MA

"Four years ago, I was at my lowest point. I was overweight, lacked energy, and felt like I was merely existing rather than truly living. That's when I discovered the incredible power of the Rainbow Diet, and it completely transformed my life. Since then, I've lost an incredible 24 pounds and regained my zest for life in ways I never thought possible.

The Rainbow Diet not only helped me shed the excess weight, but it also gave me the energy and vitality to engage in activities I had long given up on. I started hiking, biking, and even picked up playing tennis again. These were things I never imagined I would be able to enjoy, but with the Rainbow Diet, my body became lighter, stronger, and more capable. Beyond the physical benefits, the Rainbow Diet had a profound impact on my mental and emotional well-being. I became more focused and productive at work, leading to career advancements and a newfound sense of purpose. But what truly amazed me was the sense of serenity and peace that washed over me. The vibrant, nutrient-rich foods I consumed nourished not only my body but also my soul. I felt a deep connection to nature and a renewed sense of gratitude for the world around me.

The Rainbow Diet has become so much more than just a way of eating; it has become a way of life. I can't thank it enough for the incredible transformation it has brought to my life. If you're looking for a sustainable and holistic approach to wellness, I wholeheartedly recommend the Rainbow Diet. It's not just about losing weight; it's about regaining your vitality, finding joy in every moment, and unlocking your true potential."

The Rainbow Diet

—Dave J., Berkeley, CA

How to Begin—and Succeed at—the Rainbow Diet

The Rainbow Diet—and the enormous benefits it can unlock—are completely accessible to you. If you're interested in starting the Rainbow Diet, here are some helpful tips to get you started:

1. **Educate Yourself**: Familiarize yourself with the principles and guidelines of the Rainbow Diet. Learn about your chakras, the colors they are attuned to, and the energy centers and their functions in your body. The Rainbow Diet does not just guide you to eat a variety of colorful foods; it is a comprehensive system for nurturing your body, mind and spirit in a deliberate and systematic way. The cyclical pattern of nurturing each chakra, one per day, in the deliberate order from lowest to highest, puts your body into a virtuous cycle of self-care, which in turn improves your metabolism, self-confidence and inner peace.

2. **Gradual Transition**: Instead of making drastic changes overnight, start by gradually incorporating colorful foods into your diet. Many begin the Rainbow Diet with breakfast alone. It can be as simple as stocking up on fruits and berries of each color and adding them to your daily oatmeal or making a beautiful Greek yogurt and fruit parfait each morning. The Rainbow Diet is about the simplicity of nurturing each chakra in turn. You do not need to turn your life upside down to get started.

3. **Plan Your Meals**: Plan your meals in advance to ensure you have a variety of colorful ingredients on hand. Use the suggested shopping lists for ideas for the week. You can easily begin with the colorful foods you already love—but do not hesitate to expand into different or even unfamiliar foods. Mindfulness of what you are eating, and why, is an essential part of the Rainbow Diet, so allow your creativity and energy to flourish as you plan your weekly meals.

4. **Experiment with Recipes**: Explore new recipes that feature the colorful ingredients emphasized each day. This book contains numerous suggestions for different meals and snacks attuned to the correct chakra for the day—but by all means expand your horizons by trying new ideas. Many traditional foods from different cultures are centered on colorful foods, and provide a creative and exciting way to explore while improving your health and well-being.

The Rainbow Diet

5. **Mindful Eating**: Practice mindful eating by paying attention to the flavors, textures, and colors of your food. Slow down and savor each bite, appreciating the nourishment it provides to your body. When you practice the Rainbow Diet, you are literally nurturing your chakras by ingesting the energetic wavelength of that chakra in your food. But putting your focus on the day's chakra and its color also energizes that chakra, and increases the benefit your receive.

6. **Stay Hydrated**: Remember to drink plenty of water throughout the day to stay hydrated. Water helps flush out toxins and supports overall well-being. Clear, fresh water embodies and enhances every color. But you can also incorporate the day's color into your diet with teas, juices and other drinks that energize your chakras and complement your health.

7. **Listen to Your Body**: Pay attention to how different foods make you feel. Notice how the rainbow-colored foods affect your energy levels, digestion, and overall health. Adjust your diet accordingly to find what works best for you. Particularly notice how your body responds to the day's chakra. With a quick check-in several times each day, most people really notice how their hearts expand on Green Thursday (for example), and notice their increasing ability to tell their truth and use their voice on Blue Friday. You can receive immediate benefits of the Rainbow Diet by checking in with yourself and simply enjoying the enhanced state of your chakras each day.

8. **Seek Support**: Consider joining online communities or finding a support group of individuals who are also following the Rainbow Diet. Share your experiences, recipes, and tips, and seek guidance when needed.

9. **Be Brave!** It may feel like taking control of your lifestyle, diet and health can be an overwhelming step. It doesn't have to be. You can start slowly, and the Rainbow Diet will help you along your way by giving you instant results in your energy and well-being. All you need to do is take the first step.

Remember, the Rainbow Diet is not about strict rules or restrictions. It's about embracing a colorful and diverse range of whole foods that nourish your body and promote overall well-being in a structured pattern that nourishes your energy centers that creates vibrant health. Enjoy the journey and the incredible benefits that come with incorporating the vibrant spectrum of foods into your daily life and generating the virtuous cycle of the rainbow in your life.

Printed in Great Britain
by Amazon